THE BEST WAY TO ACHIEVE

Mental Holistic Wellness

is to take

"radical responsibility"

for every aspect of your

mind, body, and spiritual

well-being.

Gerard Anthony Lankester

CONTENTS

Personal Introduction

1. Understanding Holistic Wellness
2. The Body
   - The breath
   - The Gut Biome
   - The Oral Biome
   - Exercise
   - Sleep
3. Nutrition
   - Overview
   - Hydration
   - Fats
   - Sugar
   - Vitamins and Minerals
4. Looking after your body
   - Brain health
   - Diabetic health
   - Eye health
   - Heart health
   - Kidney health
   - Liver health
   - Prostate health
5. The Mind
   - Managing Emotions
   - Managing Stress
   - Developing Mindfulness
   - Building emotional resilience
   - Developing positive thought patterns

        Sharpening mental focus
        Reflections on the mind
6. The Spirit
        Embracing spiritual growth
        Culturing gratitude and mindfulness
        Journaling
        Reflections on the spirit
7. Integrating Holistic Wellness into your daily life
        General principles
        Getting down to the details
        Overcoming common challenges and obstacles
        Lack of motivation
        Time constraints
        Self-Doubt and negative self-talk
        Plateaux and setbacks
        Adapting and evolving
        Practicing self-compassion

Appendix A   My Current daily routine

GERARD ANTHONY LANKESTER

Mastering Holistic Wellness,
A Practical Guide for Every Day.

PERSONAL INTRODUCTION

I welcome you to my book, Mastering Holistic Wellness: A Practical Guide for Everyday Living.

I come to the subject with a wealth of practical life experience following a diagnosis of Bipolar Affective Disorder at the age of 54. However, I had had previous bouts of the condition probably since my teenage years and throughout my working life, unrecognised and undiagnosed. The situation became acute from the age of 50, leaving me unable to work. It resulted in several hospital stays until I reached age 60.

The epiphany moment for me was being given the diagnosis by a medical professional. This drove me to find out everything I could about the condition and how to overcome it. I researched as many books, articles, and videos on the subject as I could, I had an overwhelming drive to beat the condition and take back full control of my life. The journey also involved finding ways to master all aspects of my body, mind, and spirit. A slow process but one which lead me to a restoration of wellness from age 60. Since age 60 the progress in ever improving wellness has continued unabated. Now at the age of 71, I have been symptom free for 11 years without need for bipolar medication of any kind, and I enjoy a better quality of life, now, than ever before.

Most important of all, I have come to realise that this journey will continue for the remainder of my days on this planet. The best pathway was for me to take 'radical responsibility' for every aspect of my life. This book/guide comes with some 17 years of dedication, investigation, and personal research. I offer this book to the world as a pathway that you, the reader, can follow by taking onboard that 'radical responsibility' for yourself, too. The most important aspect of this book is that this is not a 'one size fits all' guide. It is important to apply the 'how to' tips as they apply to you now and allow your undertaking of the points to evolve and grow as you feel appropriate. For me, the essence of this book is about holistic wellness, HOW TO.

I have constructed the book with a significant number of bullet points in every chapter. These are designed to introduce you to ideas that have assisted me on my journey. If there are any points that you wish to garner further information on, I recommend that you check out the many online search engines, including Bing and Google. Much information has also been garnered from books and articles I have read over the past 17 years of research. I have also made substantial use of YouTube videos, which are a treasure trove of information for you to investigate, discover and follow up.

I have provided you with a substantial amount of information on medical issues. The reason being, I wished to highlight how you can take full proactive responsibility for any prevailing conditions you may have. I operate from a holistic wellness perspective, which, for me personally, has been and continues to be extremely beneficial. All the points I offer are from the Holistic Wellness viewpoint and are designed to complement, never replace, any advice from your healthcare professional. If you're unsure about any aspect, please use your healthcare professional as your valuable resource to complement what you seek for optimum holistic wellness.

Enjoy the journey.

MASTERING HOLISTIC WELLNESS,

A Practical Guide for Every Day.

CHAPTER 1 - UNDERSTANDING HOLISTIC WELLNESS

This book will cover the following areas:

Holistic Wellness: Understand the concept of holistic wellness, which emphasises the interconnectedness of body, mind, and spirit in achieving overall well-being. Recognise the importance of balance and harmony in all aspects of life.

1. Physical Vitality: Nurture your physical well-being through a balanced diet, regular exercise, and restful sleep. Prioritise self-care and make conscious choices that promote vitality and good health.
2. Mental Clarity: Manage stress effectively and cultivate mental clarity through mindfulness practices. Foster positive thought patterns and develop techniques to enhance focus and concentration.
3. Emotional Balance: Recognise and manage your emotions, building emotional resilience and coping mechanisms. Practice self-compassion and prioritise self-care to foster emotional well-being. Strengthen relationships and cultivate deeper emotional connections.
4. Spiritual Growth: Explore spirituality and its role in holistic wellness. Connect with nature, practice

gratitude, and develop mindfulness to nurture your spiritual well-being.
5. Integration into Daily Life: Create a personalised holistic wellness plan tailored to your lifestyle. Establish daily rituals and habits that support your well-being. Overcome challenges and obstacles on your journey and sustain long-term holistic practices for lasting benefits.

Throughout the book, you'll find practical guidance, actionable steps, and insights to help you actively engage with holistic practices and improve your overall well-being. The goal is to empower you to embrace holistic wellness in your everyday life and experience the transformative power it can have on your physical, mental, emotional, and spiritual health.

In this chapter, you will delve deeper into the concept of holistic wellness, defining its essence and exploring the principles that underpin it. By gaining a clear understanding of holistic wellness, you will be better equipped to embrace its principles and integrate them into your daily life.

Holistic wellness is an approach to well-being that recognises the interconnectedness of body, mind, and spirit. These three aspects of your being are intricately linked and influence each other in profound ways. It goes beyond focusing solely on physical health and acknowledges the importance of nurturing all dimensions of your being, including the physical, mental, emotional, and spiritual aspects. The goal of holistic wellness is to achieve a state of balance, harmony, and vitality in all areas of your life.

The Interconnectedness of Body, Mind, and Spirit:

1. The Body: Your physical body is the vessel through which you experience the world. It is important to care for your body by adopting healthy habits such as regular exercise, proper nutrition, and adequate rest. When you prioritise your physical health, you not only enhance your vitality and energy levels but also create a solid foundation for overall well-being. Physical well-being supports mental clarity, emotional stability, and spiritual growth.
2. The Mind: Your mind encompasses your thoughts, beliefs, emotions, and perceptions. It plays a significant role in your overall well-being. Your

mental state can greatly influence your physical health, as stress, anxiety, and negative thought patterns can manifest as physical ailments. By cultivating a positive and resilient mindset, practicing mindfulness, and engaging in activities that promote mental well-being, you can create a harmonious relationship between your mind and body.
3. The Spirit: The spirit refers to the essence of who you are, your innermost self, and your connection to something greater than yourself. It encompasses your values, beliefs, purpose, and sense of meaning in life. Nurturing your spiritual well-being involves exploring and deepening your connection to your inner self, engaging in practices such as meditation, contemplation, gratitude, and self-reflection. When you align with your spiritual nature, you experience a sense of purpose, inner peace, and a deeper understanding of yourself and the world around you.

Understanding the interconnectedness of body, mind, and spirit allows you to take a holistic approach to your well-being. When one aspect is out of balance, it can impact the others. For example, chronic stress can lead to physical ailments and mental exhaustion, while unresolved emotional issues can manifest as physical symptoms. By recognising and addressing these connections, you can create a harmonious synergy for the body, mind, and spirit.

Holistic practices such as yoga, tai chi, energy healing, and breathwork can help bridge the gap between these dimensions and promote their integration. These practices enhance physical health, calm the mind, and deepen your spiritual connection, fostering a state of holistic wellness.

The Importance of Maintaining Balance and Harmony for Optimal Well-being:

In this fast-paced and demanding world, it is easy to become caught up in the hustle and bustle of daily life, often neglecting the need for balance and harmony. However, maintaining equilibrium amongst the various dimensions of your life is essential for optimal well-being. Let's explore the importance of balance and harmony and discover practical strategies to cultivate them in your life.

1. Physical Balance: Your physical well-being forms the foundation for overall wellness. It is crucial to maintain a balance between activity and rest, ensuring you provide your body with the exercise and movement it needs while allowing time for rejuvenation and recovery. By listening to your body's cues and honouring your need for rest and relaxation, you can prevent burnout, reduce stress, and promote physical vitality.

2. Mental Balance: Your mental well-being plays a significant role in your overall quality of life. Balancing your mental state involves managing stress, cultivating positive thought patterns, and finding healthy ways to cope with challenges. This may involve practicing mindfulness, engaging in activities that bring you joy and relaxation, and seeking support when needed. By nurturing a balanced mindset, you enhance your ability to handle daily stressors, think clearly, and maintain emotional resilience.

3. Emotional Balance: Emotions are a natural part of being human, and maintaining emotional balance is crucial for your well-being. It involves acknowledging and expressing your emotions in healthy ways, while also cultivating emotional

resilience and inner peace. By practicing self-care, engaging in activities that bring you joy, and fostering positive relationships, you can create a harmonious emotional state that supports your overall well-being.
4. Spiritual Balance: Nurturing your spiritual well-being involves connecting with your inner self, exploring your values, and seeking meaning and purpose in life. It can be achieved through practices such as meditation, prayer, reflection, or engaging in activities that align with your core values. By fostering your spiritual connection, you tap into a source of guidance, inner peace, and a deeper sense of purpose, contributing to your overall well-being.
5. Work-Life Balance: Achieving a healthy balance between work and personal life is vital for your well-being. It involves setting boundaries, prioritising self-care, and allocating time and energy to activities that nourish your personal life and relationships. By finding a balance between your professional commitments and your personal needs, you can avoid burnout, nurture your relationships, and create a more fulfilling and harmonious lifestyle.

At the core of holistic wellness are several key principles that will guide your understanding and practice. Let's explore them now:
1. Wholeness: Holistic wellness recognises that you are a multifaceted being, and your well-being is influenced by the integration and harmony of all aspects of yourself. It emphasises the need to nurture and honour the physical, mental, emotional, and spiritual dimensions equally.
2. Interconnectedness: Holistic wellness acknowledges the interconnected nature of your

existence. It recognises that the well-being of one aspect of your life can profoundly impact other areas. For example, a healthy mind can contribute to physical well-being, and vice versa.

3. Prevention: Rather than focusing solely on treating symptoms or ailments, holistic wellness emphasises the importance of preventive care. It encourages proactive measures, such as adopting healthy lifestyle habits, managing stress, and cultivating positive relationships, to maintain overall well-being and prevent illness.
4. Personal Responsibility: Holistic wellness empowers you to take an active role in your own well-being. It recognises that you are the primary driver of your health and encourages you to make informed choices, engage in self-care practices, and take responsibility for your physical, mental, emotional, and spiritual well-being.
5. Mind-Body Connection: Holistic wellness acknowledges the intricate relationship between the mind and the body. It recognizes that your thoughts, emotions, beliefs, and attitudes can significantly impact your physical health. By cultivating positive mental and emotional states, you can enhance your overall well-being.
6. Balance: Achieving balance is a central principle of holistic wellness. It emphasises the need to find equilibrium in all areas of life, including work, leisure, activity, rest, and giving and receiving. By seeking balance, you can avoid burnout, reduce stress, and maintain a sustainable lifestyle.

Introductory Reflections

Time

1. Your time is finite, and you can never get it back. Value every moment.
2. You only get one shot at today, you have just 24 hours to make it fulfilled. Once gone it is lost forever, will you inhabit it fully? Are you living or just

existing?
3. You are the president of your life.

Self
1. Find ecstasy from within, it is not out there.
2. Practice being your best friend. 'Do unto yourself, as you would do unto others.'
3. Good habits are worth being fanatical about.

Purpose
1. Life is 10% of what happens to you and 90% of how you react to it.
2. Life without a plan leads to chaos. Avoid making life on the fly, have a plan.
3. Entertainment and distraction are the enemies of creation and learning. The fastest way to become extraordinary is to focus, learn and educate yourself. Be a lifetime learner.
4. Observe the impact of autopilot living in your habits, start by being aware. By raising awareness, you enable your power of choice, whether to continue or change.
5. Live your life with purpose, you can start with small steps that accumulate and gain momentum. Intention requires action, plan to act in small steps.
6. Action is never all or nothing. Act now not later; remember the only time to look back is to see how far you have come.

Health
1. Keeping your body healthy is an expression of gratitude to the Universe.
2. (Mahatma Gandhi) "It is health that is real wealth. And not pieces of gold and silver."
3. Be mindful of the difference between 'Lifespan' and 'Health span.' Lifespan is the total number of years that you live. People are living longer but many of

those years can be burdened by chronic diseases.
4. The aim of Mastering Holistic Wellness is to enable you to consciously take steps to optimise your Health span by living your life courageously and fulfilled, with the purpose of extending your years of healthy living, free from disease.

Now that you have a foundation in understanding holistic wellness and its principles, you can now move forward on this path, exploring the practical aspects of holistic well-being and uncovering the tools and practices that will help you master holistic wellness in your everyday life.

GERARD ANTHONY LANKESTER

Mastering Holistic Wellness, A Practical Guide for Every Day.

CHAPTER 2 - THE BODY

Let's now explore the body and see how you can impact on its efficient functioning.

The Breath

Breath - factors that can have a negative impact on your breathing.

1. Smoking or the use of tobacco products can cause respiratory problems and reduce lung capacity.
2. Exposure to second-hand smoke can irritate the airways and hinder breathing.
3. Poor indoor air quality caused by factors such as dust, pet dust, mould, or chemical pollutants, which can cause respiratory problems and hinder breathing quality.
4. Sedentary lifestyles and the lack of regular physical activity can weaken respiratory muscles and reduce lung capacity.
5. Poor posture, such as slouching or hunching, which restricts lung expansion and inhibits adequate breathing.
6. Chronic stress and anxiety, which lead to shallow breathing and affect the efficiency of oxygen exchange.
7. Environmental pollutants, such as air pollution, smoke, or industrial emissions, can irritate the

airways and compromise breathing quality.
8. Allergens such as pollen, dust mites, pet allergens can cause respiratory allergies and cause breathing problems.
9. Respiratory infections, such as colds, flu, or respiratory tract infections, can temporarily affect breathing quality and cause congestion. 10.
10. Mouth and oral diseases, such as gum disease or tooth decay, can contribute to poor breathing and affect breathing quality.
11. Dehydration, which can lead to dry mouth and reduce saliva production, resulting in bad breathing and pain during breathing.
12. Certain drugs, such as antihistamines or decongestants, can cause dryness of the respiratory system and affect breathing quality.
13. Obstructive sleep apnoea, a sleep disorder characterized by breathing interruptions during sleep, which can result in poor breath quality.
14. Acid reflux or gastroesophageal reflux disease (GERD), which can cause acid to enter the throat and affect breath quality.
15. Consuming foods and drinks that contribute to bad breath, such as onions, garlic, spicy foods, alcohol, or coffee.
16. Mouth breathing, which can lead to dry mouth, increased risk of infections, and less efficient breath intake.
17. Chronic respiratory conditions, such as asthma or chronic obstructive pulmonary disease (COPD), which can impact breath quality and lung function.
18. Environmental factors like high altitude or extreme temperatures, which can affect breath intake and respiratory function.
19. Sedatives or certain medications that depress the central nervous system, which can slow down

breathing and affect breath quality.
20. Poor indoor ventilation or working in environments with poor air circulation, which can lead to stagnant air and hinder breath quality.

Key Facts about healthy breathing

1. Breathing through your nose is healthier than through your mouth. There are more obstructions and filters through the nose to the lungs. Mouth breathing is direct into the lungs allowing viruses and infections easy access.
2. Nose breathing increases oxygen input to your lungs.
3. Nitric oxide can enter the lungs through your sinus cavity, this is good; this does not occur when mouth breathing.
4. Nose breathing long and slow increases the oxygen into your body.
5. When exercising vigorously, consciously learn to slow your breathing down to increase your oxygen assimilation. The body compensates and produces more oxygen cells to circulate through your body.
6. Check out the Wim Hoff breathing method. Empty your lungs of air and you will find your able to hold your breath for longer before the next breath intake.
7. Consciously focus on fully emptying your lungs to maximise oxygen intake into your lungs.
8. Breathing technique - 'breathe in' to a count of five, then 'breathe out' to a count of five. Then gradually extend your 'out breath' to a count of 8 or 9 or 10. N.B. The out breath is the relaxing breath.
9. Breathing exercise to lower your blood pressure - Place thumb on your left nostril, then inhale through your right nostril. N.B. This exercise also stimulates the right-hand side of your brain.

10. Breathing exercise to increase your Blood pressure - Place thumb on your right nostril then inhale through your left nostril.
11. Your nostrils can breathe through alternative sides and through both nostrils. You are then can adjust the body's physiology through the nose. This does not occur through mouth breathing.
12. Asthmatics - during an asthma attack, focus on breathing deeply through your nose and not through your mouth.
13. Anxiety and Panic - slow down your breathing and breathe through your nose. Rapid mouth breathing exacerbates your anxiety and panic. Try the 4/4/4/4 breathing method - breath into a count of 4, hold your breath to a count of 4, breathe out to a count of 4, and hold to a count of 4. Repeat as long as necessary until a feeling of calm returns. This method sends calming signals to your brain and helps to reduce anxious thoughts.
14. Shallow chest breathing through your mouth is associated with 'fight and flight' feelings.
15. Using nose breathing, focus on breathing from your stomach and make this the norm. This method enables your body diaphragm to massage your body organs.
16. Lung capacity can reduce with age - Yoga exercises can help maintain and improve your lung capacity. Take long slow breaths, this leads to increased oxygenation of your blood and reduces tension.
17. Aim to maintain your healthy breathing habit for 80% of the day.
18. What are the effects of unhealthy shallow mouth breathing? This can lead to increased inflammation in your body. This in turn can lead to increased prevalence of bugs and viruses entering your body. Nose breathing, in contrast, is

your first line of defence to counter virus attacks. Nitric oxide generated during nose breathing helps kill off bugs and blunts their impact.
19. Humming increases nitric oxide availability, 15-fold, in the blood. N.B. Nitric Oxide's bio availability lasts around four to six seconds. Hence, aim to nose breath 80% of the time.
20. The chant, "Om mani Pad me Hum" has the same six second breathing rate that mimics the body breath cycle.
21. Learn to keep your tongue on the roof of your mouth, this facilitates ease of nose breathing.
22. Tongue exercise - Keep your tongue on the roof of your palate. This strengthens your tongue muscle.
23. If you are losing your lung capacity, this can be a marker for a reducing life span. Nose breathing is all about preserving your long term health.
24. If you suffer from insomnia at night, practice the 4/4/4/4 breathing method to increase a feeling of calm.
25. Slow your breathing rate per minute through the day. Aim to breathe in and out 5 or 6 times per minute instead of 10 to 12 times per minute. This will help quieten your mind and allow space for your inner voice to speak to you.
26. Breathe and release, learn to drop adverse thoughts and actions. Use the 'out breath' as a tool to release all that is adverse. Expel all the air in your lungs on your 'out breath' - sigh if it helps.
27. Ways to increase your nitric oxide production – nose breathing, humming, via an Otto 128 tuning fork (This vibrates your bones, can activate your pituitary gland. This leads to pain relief, a sense of calm which leads to nitric oxide release. Try the tuning fork on the crown of your head, your third eye, midway behind your ears, on your cheeks near

to your ears, immediately below your cheek bone and finally the base sacrum chakra.)

28. How you breathe can be the determining factor between a panic attack and deep relaxation and calm. Not fully exhaling leads to inner anxiety.
    If you breathe in short, shallow ways or unconsciously hold your breath - resolve by taking slow deep inhalations of air through your nose with even slower and longer exhalation through your mouth.
29. Start by taking a long slow deep 'in breath' through your nose, exhale through your mouth, making the 'out breath' longer than the 'in breath.' This makes the lungs more effective by increasing relaxation and reducing stress.
30. Breathing is essential to life. It is often overlooked as a necessity for good health. Deep conscious breathing is one of the most powerful keys to enhancing physical, mental, emotional, and spiritual wellbeing.
31. Nitric oxide is a major molecule that impacts on human wellness. Elevated blood pressure can be a sign of nitric oxide deficiency. Nitric oxide relaxes blood vessels which can lead to reduced blood pressure levels.
32. Mouth wash can be bad for you if it kills off nitric oxide production. Be mindful, too, anti-biotics affect your oral biome.
33. Good dietary sources to enhance nitric oxide - dark green leafy vegetables.
34. Nitric oxide levels can decline with age but improved through a healthy whole foods diet.
35. Erectile disfunction is a vascular issue, which can be reduced through good nitric oxide levels. Nitric oxide can also help heal ulcers and bed sores for wound care.

Ways to enhance your breathing.

1. Practice deep belly breathing by inhaling slowly through your nose and allowing your abdomen to expand. Exhale fully, releasing any tension or stress.
2. Engage in regular cardiovascular exercise to strengthen your lungs and improve overall respiratory function.
3. Avoid smoking and exposure to second-hand smoke, as it can negatively impact lung health and compromise the quality of your breath.
4. Maintain good posture to allow for optimal lung expansion and proper airflow.
5. Use essential oils, such as eucalyptus or peppermint, in a diffuser to promote clear airways and enhance breath quality.
6. Practice mindful breathing techniques, such as alternate nostril breathing or box breathing, to bring awareness to your breath and promote relaxation.
7. Practice good oral hygiene by brushing your teeth and tongue regularly to reduce bacteria and promote fresh breath.
8. Stay hydrated to keep your respiratory system moist and support efficient oxygen exchange.
9. Incorporate deep breathing exercises into your daily routine, such as taking a few moments to pause and take several deep breaths before meals or during breaks.
10. Avoid exposure to air pollutants, such as outdoor pollution or indoor allergens, by using air purifiers and keeping your living environment clean.
11. Practice proper diaphragmatic breathing, focusing on expanding your lower lungs rather than shallow chest breathing.

12. Engage in activities that improve lung capacity, such as swimming or playing a wind instrument.
13. Take breaks throughout the day to step outside and breathe in fresh air.
14. Practice yoga or tai chi, which emphasise breath control and can improve respiratory function.
15. Consider using a saline nasal spray or rinse to clear nasal passages and improve breath quality.
16. Practice stress reduction techniques, such as meditation or deep relaxation exercises, as stress can impact the quality of your breath.
17. Avoid consuming foods and drinks that may contribute to bad breath, such as garlic, onions, and sugary beverages.
18. Maintain a healthy weight, as excess weight can put strain on your respiratory system and affect breath quality.
19. Improve indoor air quality by using natural cleaning products, keeping plants in your home, and opening windows for fresh air circulation.
20. Consider seeking guidance from a respiratory therapist or breathing coach who can provide personalised techniques and exercises to improve the quality of your breath intake.

In conclusion, "The only thing that stays with you from birth until death is your breath." Your breath is the total guide to living, so learn how to navigate your breath. Learn how to live, change your breath, and change your life. Go to the root, it takes longer, yet lasts a potential lifetime.

For further reading check out 'Breath' by James Nestor, an excellent read. James Nestor has also produced several YouTube videos about breath.

The Gut Biome

The gut biome, also known as the gut microbiota, refers to the diverse community of microorganisms that reside in your gastrointestinal tract, particularly the intestines. It consists of trillions of bacteria, viruses, fungi, and other microorganisms, collectively known as gut flora. The gut biome plays a crucial role in maintaining overall body wellness and is involved in various physiological processes. The gut biome interacts with the body in several ways:

1. Digestion and Nutrient Absorption: Certain bacteria in the gut biome help break down complex carbohydrates, fibre, and other nutrients that our body cannot digest on its own. They produce enzymes that aid in the digestion process and release beneficial byproducts, such as short-chain fatty acids, which provide energy to the colon cells.
2. Immune System Regulation: The gut biome plays a vital role in training and modulating the immune system. It helps distinguish between harmful pathogens and harmless substances, preventing unnecessary immune responses or allergic reactions.
3. Synthesis of Essential Nutrients: Some bacteria in the gut biome produce essential vitamins like vitamin K and certain B vitamins. These vitamins are crucial for various bodily functions, including blood clotting and energy metabolism.
4. Metabolism and Weight Regulation: The composition of the gut biome is associated with metabolic processes and body weight regulation. Certain types of bacteria may influence the extraction of calories from food and the storage of excess energy, affecting weight gain or loss.
5. Neurological Function: The gut-brain axis refers to the bi-directional communication between the gut and the brain. The gut biome plays a role in this

connection by producing neurotransmitters, such as serotonin, that can influence mood, behaviour, and mental health.

How to promote gut biome health and enhance body wellness.

1. Consuming a varied and fibre-rich diet: eating a wide range of fruits, vegetables, whole grains, and legumes provide the gut biome with diverse nutrients that support its growth and function.
2. Avoiding excessive use of antibiotics: While antibiotics are necessary in certain situations, their overuse can disrupt the balance of the gut biome by killing beneficial bacteria along with harmful ones.
3. Managing stress: Chronic stress can affect the gut-brain axis and alter the composition of the gut biome. Implementing stress-reduction techniques like meditation, exercise, and adequate sleep can help support a healthy gut.
4. Probiotic and prebiotic supplementation: Probiotics are beneficial bacteria that can be consumed through supplements or fermented foods, while prebiotics are dietary fibres that serve as food for the gut bacteria. Incorporating these into your diet can help nourish and maintain a healthy gut biome.
5. Your digestive system can store energy and looks after your five major organs, your heart, lungs, stomach, kidneys, and liver.
6. How much protein does your body require daily. Work on the following formula 0.8g of protein per kg of body weight. E.G., 87kg means 70g of protein.

By supporting a diverse and thriving gut biome, individuals can improve digestion, enhance nutrient absorption, strengthen the immune system, regulate metabolism, and promote overall body wellness.

Factors or habits that can harm the gut biome and negatively impact body wellness:

1. A poor diet rich in processed foods, refined sugar and unhealthy fats.
2. Excessive consumption of sugar beverages such as soda and fruit juice.
3. Low intake of fibre can lead to harmful imbalances in intestinal bacteria.
4. Chronic stress that may affect the axis between the intestine and the brain and affect the health of the intestine.
5. Lack of physical activity and sedentary lifestyle.
6. The excessive use or abuse of antibiotics can destroy the balance of intestinal bacteria.
7. Excessive alcohol consumption, which can damage the intestine and affect the diversity of microorganisms.
8. Smoking and tobacco consumption can have a negative impact on intestinal microbes.
9. Chronic use of non-steroidal anti-inflammatory drugs (NSAIDs) that cause intestinal inflammation.
10. Exposure to toxins and environmental pollutants.
11. Chronic sleep deprivation, which can affect the health of the intestinal tract and immune function.
12. Chronic use of protons pump inhibitors (PPIs) that alter intestinal microorganisms.
13. Chronic use of certain medications, such as steroids or immunosuppressants.
14. Digestive diseases such as Crohn's disease, ulcerative colitis, or celiac disease.
15. Food diseases or infections that disturb the intestinal microbiome.
16. Lack of diversity in diet and limited consumption of fruits, vegetables, and whole foods.

17. Artificial sweeteners, which can have a negative effect on the health of intestinal bacteria and metabolism.
18. Exposure to chronic infections such as H Pylori or parasites. Lack of appropriate hygiene practices increases the risk from harmful bacteria or viruses.
19. Lack of regular medical examination and neglect of gastrointestinal health.

Ways to improve the gut biome and optimise body wellness

1. Eat a wide variety of fruits and vegetables to ensure a wide variety of nutrients and fibres.
2. Consume fermented foods such as yogurt, sauerkraut, and Kimchi, rich in beneficial bacteria.
3. Provide prebiotic foods such as onions, garlic, leeks and bananas to feed intestinal bacteria.
4. Limit the intake of processed foods and sugar snacks that can have a negative impact on intestinal health.
5. Choose whole grains as well as brown rice, and oats, which provide fibre to gastrointestinal bacteria.
6. Drink enough water throughout the day and stay hydrated. Ideally 2 litres per day.
7. Include healthy fat sources such as avocados, nuts, seeds, that support digestive health.
8. Reduce stress levels through relaxation techniques such as meditation, deep breathing, or yoga.
9. Regular exercise to promote a healthy intestinal environment.
10. Avoid excessive use of antibiotics unless medically necessary.
11. Reduce alcohol consumption and stop smoking, as they may damage the intestines.
12. Include probiotic supplements or foods in your

daily life, such as kefir or coffee.
13. Manage your weight through a balanced diet and regular physical activity.
14. Avoid artificial sweeteners, which have a negative impact on intestinal microorganisms.
15. Get sufficient sleep to support overall health and proper digestive functions.
16. Consume adequate amounts of dietary fibre from sources like legumes, whole grains, and vegetables.
17. Limit the intake of processed meats and opt for lean sources of protein.
18. Reduce chronic inflammation through an anti-inflammatory diet rich in fruits, vegetables, and omega-3 fatty acids.
19. Practice good food hygiene to avoid foodborne illnesses that can disrupt the gut microbiota.
20. Consider talking to a healthcare professional or registered dietitian for personalised guidance and recommendations.

Incorporating these practices into your lifestyle, you can help improve the diversity and balance of your gut microbiota, leading to enhanced body wellness and overall health.

Protecting your gut biome for the over 50s

1. Nurture your gut biome with diet.
2. Improve your gut wall integrity by adding pomegranate seeds to your diet.
3. Go for a diversity of gut bacteria through pro biotic supplementation.
4. Consume specific fibres from green bananas, plantain, sprouted cashews, artichokes, chicory, asparagus, berries, hazelnuts, 70% plus dark chocolate, bone broth, and capers.
5. Take cod liver oil for health, it helps to lower heart disease risk, can improve your immunity, stamina,

joint health, and skin look. It can lower joint inflammation, stress, eye pressure from glaucoma, and appetite.
6. Eliminate, as far as possible, all sugar, stress, and tobacco.
7. Fish to avoid - all farmed fish, consume wild fish only. Avoid fish at the top of the food chain such as shark, swordfish, ocean going tuna because of mercury contamination.
8. Eat a diverse range of vegetables to optimise diversity of gut flora and depth of vitamin capture.
9. Eat soluble fibre from beans, legumes, oats, barley, berries, nuts, and seeds. Eat insoluble fibre from wheat bran, green vegetables, green beans, and whole grains.
10. Consume meat from grass fed sources rather than grain fed sources.
11. See refined carbohydrates as long-term poison and wean yourself off them as a food source.
12. Consume unpasteurised fermented foods such as kimchi, sauerkraut, kefir, and sprouted grains. N.B. Pasteurised fermented food are nowhere near as nutrient rich.

To get your gut working well, do the following.

1. Breathe into and through your stomach. This helps to reduce stress.
2. To aid digestion, chew each mouth full of food 20 times.
3. Be conscious of stomach acidity. Your stomach PH levels can decline with age. A low PH level can affect your digestion and the ability to extract the vitamins and minerals from your food. To counter this and increase your stomach acidity levels take organic apple cider vinegar, and betaine

hydrochloride supplements. Also, add lemon juice to your water. Avoid gluten, dairy, GM foods, sugar, unnecessary medicines (review with your GP), artificial colours, and preservatives.
4. Be aware of food intolerances, such as wheat and dairy. Ascertain from a qualified nutritionist which foods you are intolerant to and eliminate from your diet. Removing foods, you are intolerant to, will help to reduce body inflammation.
5. Drink warm drinks when eating food to aid stomach operation. Avoid drinking cold drinks because this can lower the quality of stomach digestion.

Mending a leaky gut

1. Tim Spector - "For great health, eat 30 different plants every week. The gut biome is contingent on the diversity of your diet."
2. Remove from your diet - highly processed foods and stress.
3. Ensure you have the right acidity PH level in your stomach.
4. Reintroduce pre and pro biotic foods, especially vegetables. Help repair your gut barrier by removing identified intolerant foods from your diet.
5. Rebalance your lifestyle by lowering your stress levels, aim for an improved work/life balance, make sleep a priority, drink water filtered to remove residual impurities, eat whole foods.
6. Fibre - aim to consume 35g of fibre daily from a diversity of different food sources.
7. Low fibre diets can allow cancer cells to proliferate.
8. Avoid foods that adversely affect the gut – e.g., sugar, highly processed grains, processed foods, alcohol, soy (only consume non-GMO soya, organic and fermented), GMO foods, dairy, unfiltered tap water,

artificial sweeteners, and frequent anti biotics.
9. Food diversity enhances the gut biome; diversity leads to resilience and stability. Eat foods in sync with the seasons.
10. H. Pylori can lead to increased blood pressure - remedies come from consuming probiotics, black seed (Nigella Sativa), broccoli sprouts, green tea, and garlic. An H. Pylori prevention food plan would include kefir, Omega 3 fatty acids, chia and flax seeds, manuka honey, berries, cruciferous vegetables, and sage. Avoid caffeine, carbonated sweet drinks, and pickled foods.
11. Foods for gut health could include red onions and purple sweet potatoes.

Highest fibre foods per 100g consumed.

1. Chia Seeds – 34g
2. Flax seeds - 27g
3. Haricot beans - 11g
4. Mixed nuts - 9g
5. Avocado, Kiwi fruit - 7 g
6. Peas, pumpkin seeds - 6g

Ways to foster a healthy gut biome.

1. Fasting helps to kill bad bugs.
2. Fibre, from whole unprocessed foods. Eat for you and your bugs.
3. Omega 3 cod liver oil.
4. Eliminate all processed seed oils. They are high in unhealthy Omega 6 and Omega 9 fats.
5. Eliminate sugar, artificial sweeteners, preservatives, emulsifiers. Read your food labels during your food shopping.
6. Aim for 7 to 8 hours of quality sleep per night. Remember, your gut has its own circadian rhythm,

too!
7. Manage stress through meditation, yoga, breath control.
8. Regular exercise - increases body levels of butyrate which improves blood vessel condition and gut flora.
9. Reduce polyps in the colon through eating foods such as sauerkraut, kimchi, kefir, bone broth (increases glutamine in your system, found in fish and meat), garlic, organic apple cider vinegar, herbs, and spices (such as turmeric, ginger, and basil).
10. Food is no longer a 'one size fits all', your gut biome is unique to you. Check out the Zoe Glucose Monitoring system. See a nutritionist to establish your food intolerances and thereby minimise potential inflammation in your body.
11. A serious thought - If you are unwilling to eat something you put on your skin - don't put it on your body! Beware phthalates, they have been identified as endocrine disrupting chemicals that interfere with hormonal actions. Phthalates are also found in some foods we eat.
12. If your arm pits are puffed rather than pitted, this can indicate your body is slow in eliminating body toxins. N.B. Deodorants can block this elimination.
13. Maintain your muscle mass into old age for longevity. Remember muscle loss can create insulin resistance. To counter, lift weights to build muscle. Cardio exercises are good for mental health, not though for gaining muscle.

The Oral Biome

(Dr Liao) "You are the owner/operator of your mouth and the CEO of your health."

What is the Oral Biome and how does it work in creating body wellness? The oral biome, also known as the oral microbiome, refers to the complex ecosystem of microorganisms that reside in the mouth. It consists of bacteria, viruses, fungi, and other microbes that interact with each other and the host (our bodies) in various ways. The oral biome plays a crucial role in maintaining oral health and has implications for overall body wellness.

The oral biome performs the following important functions:

1. Digestion: Some bacteria in the oral biome help break down food particles, initiating the digestion process before it reaches the stomach.
2. Protection: Beneficial bacteria in the oral biome help protect against harmful pathogens by competing for resources and producing antimicrobial substances.
3. Immune system support: The oral biome interacts with the immune system, helping to educate and regulate immune responses in the mouth and beyond.
4. Dental health: The oral biome influences oral health by promoting a balanced pH, preventing tooth decay, and reducing the risk of gum disease.
5. Systemic health: Emerging research suggests that imbalances in the oral biome may contribute to various systemic health conditions, including cardiovascular disease, diabetes, respiratory infections, and even certain cancers.

To promote a healthy oral biome and support overall body wellness, it's important to adopt good oral hygiene practices.

1. Only you can maintain a healthy mouth environment, it is your responsibility to keep your mouth environment alkaline rather than acidic. Your gut and oral biome are connected via your

saliva. Grow good bacteria for your oral biome, this positively impacts your sinuses, gums, teeth, and ultimately your whole body.
2. Brush your teeth twice a day using a quality toothpaste.
3. Flossing daily to remove plaque and debris between teeth.
4. Using an antimicrobial mouthwash or natural alternatives like oil pulling.
5. Eating a balanced diet, rich in fruits, vegetables, and whole foods, while limiting sugary acidic foods and beverages.
6. Avoiding tobacco products and excessive alcohol consumption.
7. Regularly visiting your dentist for check-ups and professional cleanings.

By maintaining a healthy oral biome, you can support not only your dental health but also contribute to your overall well-being.

Bad habits that can harm the oral biome and impact body wellness:

1. Bad oral hygiene practices, such as infrequent brushing and flossing.
2. Consuming excessive amounts of sugar, acidic foods and beverages.
3. Smoking and the use of tobacco products can increase the risk of gum disease and oral cancer.
4. Use of other non-smoking tobacco products.
5. Excessive alcohol consumption causes dry mouth and increases the risk of oral infections.
6. Daily snacks, especially sugary or sticky foods.
7. Neglecting regular dental examinations and professional cleaning.
8. Ignoring oral problems such as decay of teeth or

gum disease, allowing it to aggravate over time.
9. The tooth-grazing can lead to enamel erosion and damage to oral tissues.
10. The use of toothbrushes with hard bristles, which can cause gum irritation and enamel wear.
11. Use of inappropriate brushing techniques, such as aggressive brushing or excessive force.
12. Sharing toothbrushes and other oral hygiene tools that can transmit harmful oral bacteria.
13. Use of obsolete or outdated oral care products.
14. The excessive use of antibacterial oral mouthwashes, which disturbs the natural balance of oral microorganisms.
15. Ignoring the relationship between oral health and general health, ignoring oral health problems that may eventually affect your body.
16. Using certain medications that can cause dry mouth as a side effect, reducing saliva flow and impacting the oral microbiome.
17. Having a diet low in essential nutrients and vitamins needed for oral and overall health.
18. Experiencing chronic stress, which can contribute to oral health problems like teeth grinding and gum disease.
19. Suffering from certain medical conditions that can affect oral health, such as diabetes or autoimmune disorders.
20. Engaging in high-risk activities without proper protection, such as contact sports without wearing a mouthguard.

By being aware of these potential harms and making conscious efforts to avoid or mitigate them, you can help protect the oral biome and promote better oral health and overall wellness.

Controlling dental plaque

1. Avoid all sugars, they make your mouth acidic, a breeding ground for plaque and eventually tooth decay.
2. Create your own mouth wash - using 2 level teaspoons of Xylitol, 1 level teaspoon of food grade bicarbonate of soda and mixed with 5 drops of peppermint oil mix with a cup of water. Gargle and do not swallow.
3. Sesame seeds chew seeds for two minutes, then brush teeth, follow by rinsing mouth with water. Do not swallow the seeds.
4. Sip water mixed with apple cider vinegar.
5. Cloves help kill mouth bacteria.
6. Hard cheese is alkaline for the mouth.
7. Apples, figs, and spicy foods help to stimulate the saliva glands.

Ways to counter receding gums.

1. Use a soft bristle toothbrush.
2. Daily gargle of your mouth with warm salt water.
3. Tea tree oil on your toothbrush, massage your teeth and gums gently.
4. Drink lemon water daily.
5. Drink green tea.
6. Floss your teeth daily.
7. Use 'Te Pe' brushes to remove food debris from between your teeth. Cold pressed sesame oil with clove oil (rinse for up to 20 minutes daily).
8. Eliminate sugar from your diet.
9. Low carbohydrate food plan. Avoid starchy carbohydrates.

Avoid negative tooth products and chemicals. They disrupt the balanced oral micro biome.

1. Sodium lauryl sulphate

2. Sodium fluoride
3. Triclosan
4. Artificial colour dyes (from coal tar)
5. Diethanolamine
6. Microbeads
7. Artificial sweeteners
8. Any toothpastes with silica, they can strip away tooth enamel.
9. Mouth washes with alcohol
10. Minimise your stress, stress reduces mouth saliva and increases mouth acidity.
11. Too much salt can dry your mouth.

Repopulate your mouth with healthy oral flora that are complimentary for oral health.

1. Repopulate your mouth with healthy oral flora that are complementary to your oral health. Lactobacillus reuteri
2. Lactobacillus
3. Biobacteriumlactis (helps improve the closure of gum pockets)
4. Salivarius A2 5. Salivarius B (Helps remove tooth stains)
5. B lactis BL-04 (to ensure a balanced gut and mouth bacteria)
6. Inulin (strongly supports a good balance of bacteria)
7. Malic acid (from strawberries) for the coloration of teeth.
8. Dicalcium phosphate (calcium for your teeth)
9. Peppermint for freshness of breathing. All come in the form of sugar-free dental gum. These beneficial qualities are released in the mouth and are not destroyed by stomach acid.

Ways to improve the oral biome and optimise body wellness:

1. Brush your teeth thoroughly at least twice a day with a soft bristle toothbrush and fluoride toothpaste.
2. Floss daily to remove plaque and food waste from between your teeth.
3. Use anti-microbial mouth wash or with saltwater to help control harmful bacteria.
4. Clean your tongue with a tongue brush or brush to remove bacteria and prevent bad breath.
5. Avoid sugar-containing foods and beverages as they can contribute to tooth decay and disturb oral health.
6. Eat a balanced diet rich in fruits, vegetables, whole grains, and lean proteins, which provide essential nutrients for oral and overall health.
7. Limit the intake of processed foods, snacks and beverages that can promote the growth of harmful bacteria.
8. Drink lots of water throughout the day to maintain saliva production and oral health.
9. Sugar free chewing gum and mints that contain xylitol can help stimulate saliva flow and reduce the risk of tooth decay.
10. Avoid tobacco products, as they can damage oral tissues and disrupt oral bacteria.
11. Practice stress management techniques, as stress can affect oral health and the balance of the oral microorganisms.
12. Consider using probiotic supplements or eating probiotic-rich foods such as kefir and fermented foods to promote a healthy oral microbiome.
13. Maintain good overall health, as systemic conditions like diabetes and immune disorders can impact the oral biome.
14. Practice good oral hygiene habits from an early age

and teach children the importance of oral care.
15. Avoid excessive alcohol consumption, as it can contribute to dry mouth and negatively impact oral health.
16. Use a mouthguard during sports or activities that may pose a risk of dental injuries.
17. Avoid using your teeth as tools to open packages or bite into hard objects to prevent tooth fractures and damage to the oral tissues.
18. Clean and replace your toothbrush regularly to prevent the accumulation of bacteria.
19. Get regular dental check-ups and professional cleanings to maintain oral health and address any issues promptly.
20. Discuss any oral health concerns or changes with your dentist or healthcare provider to receive appropriate guidance and treatment.

Incorporating these practices into your daily routine, you can improve the health of your oral biome and promote overall body wellness.

Exercise

Incorporating regular exercise and movement into your daily routine is a key aspect of improving and maintaining your physical well-being. Exercise offers a multitude of benefits that go beyond just physical fitness. It boosts your energy levels, enhances mood, promotes better sleep, and strengthens your overall resilience.

1. Find Activities You Enjoy: Discover physical activities that bring you joy and fulfilment. Whether it's jogging, dancing, swimming, yoga, or team sports, finding activities you genuinely enjoy increases the likelihood of sticking to a regular exercise routine.
2. Set Realistic Goals: Establish realistic goals that

align with your current fitness level and overall health. Start with achievable targets and gradually progress over time. This approach helps prevent injury and keeps you motivated as you witness your progress.
3. Mix Up Your Routine: Keep your exercise routine diverse and engaging by incorporating different types of activities. This not only prevents boredom but also allows you to work different muscle groups, improve overall strength and flexibility, and maintain overall interest in your fitness journey.
4. Prioritise Consistency: Consistency is key when it comes to exercise. Aim for regular physical activity, even if it's in shorter durations. Consistency builds habits and makes it easier to maintain an active lifestyle in the long run.
5. Make It a Daily Habit: Find opportunities to include movement throughout your day, even outside of dedicated exercise sessions. Take the stairs instead of the elevator, go for a walk during your lunch break, or engage in active hobbies such as gardening or dancing. These small bursts of activity add up and contribute to your overall well-being.
6. Listen to Your Body: Pay attention to your body's signals and adjust your exercise routine accordingly. Rest when needed, and don't push yourself beyond your limits. It's essential to find a balance between challenging yourself and giving your body the time, it needs to recover and repair.
7. Seek Variety and Progression: As you become comfortable with your routine, challenge yourself by increasing the intensity, duration, or complexity of your workouts. This progressive approach helps prevent plateauing and keeps your body continually adapting and improving.
8. Stay Motivated: Find sources of motivation that

resonate with you. Set rewards for achieving fitness milestones, exercise with a friend or join a group class for added accountability and support or track your progress using fitness phone apps or wearable devices. Remember that each step you take towards better physical well-being is an achievement worth celebrating.

How to incorporate exercise into your daily routine:

1. Start with Morning Stretches: Begin your day with gentle stretches to awaken your body and prepare it for the day ahead. Spend a few minutes stretching major muscle groups, focusing on areas that feel tight or tense.
2. Take Active Breaks: Break up long periods of sitting or desk work by incorporating short bursts of physical activity. Set a timer to remind yourself to stand up, stretch, or take a brisk walk around the office or your home.
3. Walk Whenever Possible: Opt for walking instead of driving for short distances. Park your car farther away from your destination, take the stairs instead of the elevator, or get off public transportation one stop earlier and walk the remaining distance.
4. Make Use of Technology: Utilise fitness apps or wearable devices to track your daily steps and set activity goals. These tools can provide motivation and reminders to keep moving throughout the day.
5. Schedule Exercise Time: Treat exercise as important as your diary appointments by scheduling it into your daily calendar. Set aside dedicated time for activities such as jogging, cycling, swimming, or attending fitness classes. Consistency is key, so make it a non-negotiable part of your routine.
6. Combine Exercise with Daily Tasks: Find creative

ways to incorporate exercise into your daily tasks. For example, while doing household chores, add extra movements like lunges, squats, or calf raises. Turn mundane tasks into opportunities for physical activity.
7. Involve Others: Engage in physical activities with friends, family, or colleagues. Join a sports team, go for group walks, or participate in fitness challenges together. Having a social aspect to your exercise routine can make it more enjoyable and help maintain your motivation.
8. Explore Active Hobbies: Discover activities or hobbies that involve movement and align with your interests. Whether it's dancing, gardening, hiking, or practicing martial arts, finding enjoyable activities increases the likelihood of sticking to them in the long term.
9. Make TV Time Active: Instead of sitting idly while watching TV, use the time to engage in light exercises. Perform bodyweight exercises, use resistance bands, or do yoga or Pilates routines while enjoying your favourite shows.
10. Prioritise Rest and Recovery: Remember that rest and recovery are essential for maintaining overall physical well-being. Allow yourself time to rest and recharge between exercise sessions to prevent burnout and injury.

Every little bit of physical activity counts, and even small changes can have a significant impact on your overall physical well-being.

Training for health and longevity

1. Take regular aerobic training, choose what best interests you personally, this can be in the form of individual exercises or group activities or a

combination of the two types. Exercises can include walking, running, endurance training, high impact interval training.

2. Enjoy regular sleep patterns, sleep is essential for quality of life, and it is the primary method by which your brain can assimilate your activities during the previous time since your last sleep. Aim for quality sleep and a regular duration of at least 7 to 8 hours a night. Modern applications on your phone or smart watch can monitor these key elements. Monitor the duration of your sleep, as well as the quality - be aware of the ratio between light sleep, deep sleep, and REM sleep.

3. Eat like your ancestors consuming whole foods only, avoid fake highly processed food.

4. Walk barefoot on the earth for earthing with the planet earth. This assists in reducing body inflammation and improving your circadian rhythms. Earthing mats can mimic the process of walking barefoot.

5. Drink clean clear water. A water filter is appropriate to eliminate water impurities. In addition, store water in glass containers rather than plastic. This avoids contamination from plastic nano particles.

6. Useful sources of exercising, body building (to increase body muscle and in later life to maintain muscle mass), powerlifting, cross fit training, cardio exercising (hiking, brisk walking, cycling, running), yoga, and meditation amongst many others.

7. Important exercises for the over 50s include squats, wall sliding, stretching, and stepping. These exercises help to improve balance and poise.

What are the benefits of regular exercising?

1. Benefits your sympathetic and parasympathetic

systems.
2. Helps reduce the risk of heart disease. Exercise helps increase the variability of heart rate and leads to an increase in overall body strength.
3. Helps to reduce the risk of high blood pressure.
4. Helps reduce the risk of stroke.
5. Helps reduce the risk of cancer.
6. Helps to reduce the risk of diabetes by increasing insulin sensitivity.
7. Helps to reduce the risk of anxiety and depression.
8. Helps reduce the risk of dementia.
9. Helps to reduce stress feelings.
10. Helps reduce inflammation in the body.
11. Helps reduce lower back pain.
12. Exercise helps to improve your mental will power.
13. Exercise can improve and increase longevity.
14. Exercise can improve fertility.
15. Exercise can increase body energy.

How to increase muscle in the body

1. Time under tension - try 60 seconds of slow tension. This consists of 20 seconds on the rise, followed by 20 seconds of holding, then 20 seconds on the descend.
2. Never starve yourself of food.
3. Include days without carbohydrates, low carbohydrates, and high carbohydrates; this approach allows you to maintain your metabolism and reduce surplus fat reserves.
4. For two or three days a week, you conduct a 15-minute high-intensity impact training (HIIT) in the exercise of your choice. HIIT targets fat cells due to its afterburn effect.

Some HIIT exercises

1. Squats - 60 seconds, an important exercise for balance.
2. Push ups - 30 seconds
3. Mountain climber plank, touch the floor with alternate legs - 30 seconds.
4. Lunges, step forward knee hitting the floor then alternate with the other knee - 60 seconds.
5. Brisk walking to lose weight - 100 calories to about 2000 steps. The 2000 steps are equivalent to approximately 1 mile.

Running, tips for running longer distances

1. Start slowly, if you are breathless, you are running too fast for your aerobic system.
2. Your pace should be "breathe in" for 3 steps and "breathe out" for 3 steps.
3. Run more frequently.
4. Focus on your form and remember that your posture is important.
5. When you feel that your legs are heavy, focus your attention on your arms.
6. Start with a stop at 1, 2, and 3km in your 4 km route. Reduce your stops until you can finish your run without stopping.
7. Running the terrain - Running the flat and sloped terrain and walking up hill
8. Walk uphill but never stop,
9. Start running slowly and gradually increase your pace.
10. Run with someone or listen to music. Engage in positive thinking and self-confidence.

Sleep

A good night's sleep is essential for optimising wellness, so 7 to 8 hours of sleep every night is essential. Not only is time sleeping important but also the quality of your sleep, namely the ratio of light sleep, deep sleep, and REM sleep. Use a smart watch and/or a sleep monitoring phone application to enable you to keep abreast of your sleep quality.

Here are some practical ways strategies to enhance sleep quality and promote restful sleep on a day-to-day basis.

1. Establish a Bedtime Routine: Create a consistent bedtime routine that prepares your body and mind for sleep. Engage in relaxing activities like reading a book, listening to calming music, or practicing gentle stretches. This routine will signal to your brain that it's time to unwind and prepare for rest.
2. Maintain a Regular Sleep Schedule: Aim to go to bed and wake up at the same time every day, even at weekends. This helps regulate your body's internal clock and promotes a natural sleep-wake cycle. Consistency in your sleep schedule will improve sleep quality and make it easier to fall asleep and wake up refreshed.
3. Create a Sleep-Friendly Environment: Ensure your sleep environment is comfortable and conducive to restful sleep. Keep your bedroom dark, quiet, and at a cool temperature. Use blackout curtains, earplugs, or a white noise machine to block out any disruptive sounds or light that may interfere with your sleep.
4. Limit Exposure to Electronic Devices: Minimise exposure to electronic devices, such as smartphones, tablets, and TVs, especially before bedtime. The blue light emitted by these devices can suppress the production of melatonin, a hormone that regulates sleep. Instead, engage in relaxing activities like reading a physical book or practicing relaxation techniques.

5. Manage Stress and Anxiety: Develop strategies to manage stress and anxiety, as these can significantly impact your sleep quality. Prioritise stress reduction techniques such as deep breathing exercises, meditation, or journaling before bed. This will help calm your mind and promote a more peaceful state for sleep.
6. Create a Sleep-Friendly Routine: Establish a pre-sleep routine that signals to your body that it's time to wind down. This could involve taking a warm bath or shower, practicing gentle yoga, or stretching, or sipping a soothing herbal tea like chamomile. Consistently engaging in these activities before bed will help cue your body for sleep.
7. Avoid Stimulants and Heavy Meals: Limit your intake of stimulants such as caffeine and nicotine, particularly in the afternoon and evening. These substances can interfere with your ability to fall asleep. Additionally, avoid spicy, or large meals close to bedtime, as they can cause discomfort and disrupt your sleep.
8. Create a Relaxing Sleep Environment: Make your bedroom a sanctuary for sleep. Invest in a comfortable mattress, pillows, and bedding that support your sleep needs. Experiment with different sleep aids like essential oils, calming scents, or a comfortable eye mask to enhance relaxation and create a soothing sleep environment.

Sleep awareness strategies

1. 80% to 90% of serotonin is produced in the gut. Serotonin is the seed that helps produce melatonin for sleep. There is around 400 times more melatonin in your gut than your brain. Thus, your

gut microbiome has a huge impact on your sleep.
2. Avoid all processed foods and drinks.
3. Avoid haphazard use of antibiotics.
4. Beware of pesticides, heavy metals, acid blockers.
5. Eat fermented foods such as kefir, sauerkraut, and kimchi.
6. Some nutrients which aid sleep are vitamin C rich foods, iron, calcium (Greens, tahini, tinned oily fish), Omega 3 fats, and magnesium.
7. Reduce blue light radiation after dark from your TV, phone, computer, and tablet. They suppress melatonin.
8. Switch off your Wi-Fi at night or install a Wi-Fi timer.
9. Minimise the amount of electrical magnetic radiation from electrical devices in your bedroom. Unplug them if necessary.
10. Meditation aids your sleep cycle.
11. Last thing, before sleep, review your day and what you wish to achieve the following day.
12. Put a pillow under your ankles to aid lymphatic clear out. When sleeping, keep your head at a lower level than your ankles.
13. When travelling internationally, preserve your sleeping window. Avoid eating during your sleeping window. This is especially important when travelling by aero plane and crossing time zones. This will ensure you do not disrupt your circadian rhythms. Avoid all carbohydrates on an airflight.

GERARD ANTHONY LANKESTER

Mastering Holistic Wellness,
A Practical Guide for Every Day.

CHAPTER 3 - THE BODY – NUTRITION

Nutrition Overview

Discover the vital role that nutrition plays in achieving holistic wellness and unlock the key to a balanced and wholesome diet. In this exploration, "Mastering Holistic Wellness: A Practical Guide for Every Day" dives deep into the profound connection between what you consume and your overall well-being.

Learn here how to make informed choices about your diet and harness the transformative power of nutrition.

1. You will discover the secrets of nourishing your body with the right fuel it craves for optimum performance and vitality.
2. Learn how to strike a harmonious balance between macronutrients and micronutrients, embracing whole foods that nourish you from the inside out.
3. Discover the profound impact of superfoods, herbs, and supplements that enhance your body's natural healing capabilities.
4. Uncover practical tips to cultivate a healthy relationship with food, addressing emotional eating, stress-related eating patterns, and mindful food choices.
5. Above all, find joy and satisfaction in nourishing yourself.
6. Empower yourself with the knowledge and tools to

create a balanced and wholesome diet that supports your holistic well-being.
7. Embrace Whole Foods: Focus on incorporating whole, unprocessed foods into your diet. Fill your plate with a colourful variety of fruits, vegetables, whole grains, lean proteins, and healthy fats. Nutrient-rich foods provide essential vitamins, minerals, and antioxidants to support your overall well-being.
8. Portion Control: Practice mindful portion control to maintain a balanced diet. Pay attention to your body's hunger and fullness cues and aim for appropriate serving sizes.
9. Avoid oversized portions. And opt for smaller plates to help regulate your food intake.
10. Balance Macronutrients: Include a balance of macronutrients – carbohydrates, proteins, and fats – in your meals. Carbohydrates provide energy, proteins support muscle growth and repair.
11. Fats aid in nutrient absorption.
12. Opt for complex carbohydrates, lean proteins, and unsaturated fats for a well-rounded diet.
13. Mindful Eating: Cultivate a mindful eating practice by slowing down and savouring each bite. Pay attention to the flavours, textures, and sensations of the food you consume. This practice enhances your connection with food, promotes better digestion, and helps prevent overeating.
14. Plan and Prepare: Take time to plan and prepare your meals in advance. This helps you make healthier choices and reduces reliance on processed or fast foods. Set aside a dedicated time each week to meal planning, grocery shopping, and meal prepping to ensure you have nourishing options readily available.
15. Listen to Your Body: Tune in to your body's signals

and honour its unique needs. Pay attention to how different foods make you feel. Experiment with an intuitive eating approach when you eat.
16. Based on your body's hunger and fullness cues rather than rigid external rules.
17. Remember, achieving a balanced and wholesome diet is a lifelong journey. It's about nourishing your body with nutrient-dense foods while finding joy and satisfaction in the eating experience.
18. Seek Professional Guidance: Consult a registered dietitian or nutritionist for personalised advice and guidance. They can help tailor a diet plan that meets your specific dietary needs, health goals, and any underlying conditions or food intolerances you may have.

With a mindful approach and a commitment to your well-being, you can embrace a balanced diet that supports your holistic wellness goals.

Hydration

Hydration is Key: Stay hydrated by drinking an adequate amount of water throughout the day. Water plays a crucial role in digestion, nutrient absorption, and overall body function. Limit sugary beverages and prioritise water as your primary choice of hydration.

Fats

Fat is essential to a healthy diet as it gives us energy and helps our bodies absorb vitamins and nutrients from the foods we eat. However, fats contain more calories than carbohydrates and protein so it's important to limit how much you consume. Eating too much fat too often can lead to weight gain and other health problems.

Unsaturated fats

Unsaturated fats can help to lower your blood cholesterol, reducing your risk of developing heart disease. They also provide your body with essential fatty acids, important for keeping your muscles, skin, and other tissue healthy. These types of fats are found in:
1. Oily fish - such as mackerel and salmon
2. Avocados
3. Nuts and seeds.
4. Plant-based oils and spreads - such as olive and rapeseed.

Saturated and trans-fats

These raise the level of cholesterol in your blood, increasing your risk of developing heart disease. You'll benefit from reducing your intake of these type of fats. Saturated fats are found in:
1. Processed meat products - such as sausages and beef burgers.
2. Butter and lard.
3. Full-fat cream, milk, and ice-cream
4. Hard cheese - such as parmesan and cheddar
5. Biscuits, cakes, and pastries.

Current UK government guidelines recommend that:

1. Men should eat 95g of fat (30g of saturates) in their diet each day.
2. Women should eat 70g of fat (20g of saturates) in the diet each day.

Sugar

Sugar is a carbohydrate that provides the body with energy. Some foods naturally contain sugar – such as fruit, vegetables, wholegrains, and dairy foods. Other foods have sugar added to them in the manufacturing process. These are called free or added sugars. Free sugars are found in:

1. Sweets and chocolate.
2. Sugary drinks.
3. Cakes and puddings.
4. Ice cream
5. Breakfast cereals
6. Flavoured yoghurts

They're also naturally present in:
1. Syrups
2. Honey
3. Fruit juices

Most of us eat too many food products containing free sugars. Ideally, no more than 5% of the energy we consume should come from free sugars. Currently, children and adults across the UK are consuming 2 to 3 times this amount.

Current UK Government guidelines recommend that:

1. Adults should have a maximum of 30g (roughly 7.5 teaspoons) of free sugar a day.
2. Children aged 7 to 10 years – 24g (roughly 6 teaspoons)
3. Children aged 4 to 6 years – 19g (roughly 4.75 teaspoons)

Cutting down on free sugar

1. Sugary drinks account for a surprisingly large proportion of the daily sugar intake of both children and adults. Almost a third of the free sugars consumed by 11- to 18-year-olds come from soft drinks.
2. Foods that contain free sugars aren't required as part of a healthy balanced diet, so you should try to eat these less often and in smaller amounts.
3. To do this, use food labels to choose items that are lower in sugar and swap:
4. Switch sugary breakfast cereals for plain cereals –

such as plain porridge, wholewheat biscuit cereals, shredded wholewheat or no added sugar muesli.
5. Switch flavoured or corner-style yoghurts for low sugar yoghurts, adding fresh fruit for variety.
6. Switch sugary drinks for water, lower fat milk, sugar-free drinks or tea and coffee.
7. Cereal bars often contain high levels of free sugars too, so remember to check the label.

Weight gain

1. Sugar is easy to consume in large quantities as it's pleasant to taste. This means many people eat too much sugar and get more calories than they need.
2. If you consume more calories than your body needs, your body stores the energy as glycogen or fat in your liver, muscles, and fat cells to use later. This can lead to weight gain.
3. To prevent weight gain, and an increased risk of health problems like type 2 diabetes, reduce the amount of sugar in your diet overall. You should get most of the energy you need from unprocessed starchy foods (potatoes, brown rice, pasta, and whole grain cereals) without the need to eat free sugars.

Tooth decay

1. When you eat sugar, the bacteria in your mouth produce acid. This acid dissolves the enamel on your teeth, causing tooth decay and cavities to form.
2. Eat fewer sugary foods that stick to your teeth – such as sweets and dried fruits.
3. Eat fewer sugary snacks between meals.
4. Swap for sugar-free drinks – such as water or milk.
5. Only consume foods and drinks containing sugar at mealtimes.

6. Sugars found naturally in fruits, vegetables and dairy are less likely to cause tooth decay.
7. However, fruit juices contain a lot of sugar so should only be consumed at mealtimes.

For more about preventing tooth decay – see Chapter 2 The Body – The Oral biome.

For individual foods, you can verify their nutritional values by logging onto any of the big supermarket phone applications or online.

When it comes to nutrition, it is best to keep a log of your food intake, there are several excellent food logging phone applications, some are free, some require a subscription after a free period. Using these applications enable you to keep a 'finger on the pulse' of your food intake. Nutracheck and MyNetDiary are particularly helpful examples.

An overview of the importance of Vitamins and Minerals from your Food intake.

Vitamins and minerals are essential nutrients that your body needs in small amounts to work properly. People should be able to get all the nutrients they need by eating a varied and balanced diet. If you choose to take vitamin and mineral supplements, seek advice where appropriate.

Fat-soluble vitamins

1. Fat-soluble vitamins (vitamin A, D, E and K) are mainly found in:
2. Animal fats
3. Vegetable oils
4. Dairy foods
5. Liver
6. Oily fish
7. While your body needs these vitamins to work properly, you don't need to eat foods containing

them every day.

Water-soluble vitamins

Water-soluble vitamins (vitamin C, the B vitamins and folic acid) are mainly found in:
1. Fruit and vegetables
2. Grains
3. Milk and dairy foods

These vitamins aren't stored in the body, so you need to have them more frequently. If you have more than you need, your body gets rid of the extra vitamins when you urinate.

Minerals

Minerals include calcium and iron amongst many others and are found in:
1. Meat
2. Wholegrain cereals.
3. Fish
4. Milk and dairy foods.
5. Fruit and vegetables.
6. Nuts and seeds.

Minerals are necessary for 3 main reasons:
1. Building strong bones and teeth
2. Controlling body fluids inside and outside your cells
3. Turning the food, you eat, into energy.

Trace elements

1. Trace elements are also essential nutrients that your body needs to work properly, but in much smaller amounts than vitamins and minerals. They include iodine and fluorine.
2. Trace elements are found in small amounts in a variety of foods such as meat, fish, cereals, milk and dairy foods, vegetables, and nuts.

Mastering Holistic Wellness,
A Practical Guide for Every Day.

CHAPTER 4 - THE BODY – LOOKING AFTER YOUR BODY.

Brain Health

Here are some suggestions to help you enhance your brain health.

1. Be aware of being nutrient deficient from a poor diet.
2. Avoid sugar. Be mindful of the impact of sugar has on your body. Excessive sugar is a poison and can lead to a leaky gut, insulin resistance, and Altheimer's disease.
3. Avoid vegetable seed oils, and all processed foods.
4. Limit excessive intake of starchy carbohydrates.
5. Limit caffeine intake.
6. Be aware of wheat intolerance. The best grains to consume are whole grains so avoid processed grains.
7. Improve gut health, remove environmental toxins from the body, e.g., lead and mercury.
8. Reducing the impact of autism. Investigate gut issues, balance of good and bad bugs in the gut, low vitamin levels arising from poor absorption of nutrients and/poor dietary choices.
9. For Alzheimer's, consider the gut system. Are levels of Vitamin B1, B6, and B12 adequate, check

MASTERING HOLISTIC WELLNESS

homocysteine levels.
10. Establish, via a food intolerance test, your food, and hormone sensitivities. Check out continuous glucose monitoring to establish how your body works.
11. Be wise to body inflammation arising from food intolerances, processed foods, and insulin resistance.
12. Sleep apnoea affects the quality of your sleep and your brain's repair function. Sleep apnoea is exacerbated by being overweight. Address your breath issues by avoiding mouth breathing, instead, get in the habit of nose breathing.
13. Be the CEO of your health, take radical responsibility for it. When shopping read the food labels, if the ingredients are unknown or not normally stored in your food cupboard – avoid.
14. Assist your brain health with whole foods, exercise, high intensity impact training, sleep, (to reduce stress), take up meditation and yoga.
15. Regarding supplements – check out quality of your diet, sleeping patterns, exercise, quality of the gut biome. If poor absorption from food, consider supplementing with B Vitamins, Vitamin D3, and Magnesium.
16. Amongst the top foods for brain health are fatty fish, avocado, nuts and seeds, olive oil, eggs, berries, leafy greens, turmeric, and green tea.
17. Coenzyme Q10 assists brain function and is needed for processing B Vitamins in the body.
18. Align your body to your circadian rhythms for health and wellness.
19. Cold showers increase the good 'brown fat' stores. Probiotic foods are great gut health additions e.g., cranberries, pomegranates, berries, and green tea.
20. Intermittent fasting is great for long term health,

enabling the disposal of weak and dead cells and replacing them with new vigorous cells.

Bipolar Affective disorder

1. Manic symptoms - mania, unusually happy and intensely so. No need for sleep. Very fast talking from racing thoughts, restless, easily distracted, delusional, excessive over confidence, risky behaviours (including excessive spending, sex, alcohol, substance abuse, gambling), inability to complete tasks, aggression, irritability. Increasingly unhealthy diet.
2. Depression symptoms – depression, uncontrollable sadness, helplessness, obsession with negative thoughts, noise sensitivity, withdrawal from family and friends, isolating ignoring phone calls and messages, agoraphobia, losing all interest in activities you previously enjoyed, major fatigue, low energy, sleeping for very long hours, slow talking, unfocused, quieter, poor memory, physical pain, lack of hygiene, feelings of being stuck forever, bottomless pit of desperation and despair, an inability to experience pleasure which can last for months, ideation of ending life through suicide.

In all cases seek urgent medical assistance.

How to avoid digital overload and enhance brain health.

1. To avoid list – Multi tasking, being at the beck and call of your phone every day, (excess phone use lowers attention span, fosters distraction and reactivity).
2. To embrace list – Switch off your phone daily, put in silent mode, do not use for periods during the day e.g., for first hour after waking, for at least one hour

before sleep, put in bag or in your pocket in silent mode when out walking.
3. Take cold showers each morning, embrace meditation, set yourself 3 personal and 3 professional goals to complete daily.
4. Digital overload arises from low dopamine sensitivity – leads to overdoing and encourages the brain to obtain the easy stimulation it craves. Think of Dopamine as '<u>digital heroin</u>'.

Lower your cancer risk.

1. Cancer cells feed off sugar. Cancer cells hate oxygen whilst healthy cells love oxygen. Glucose and glutamine feed cancer cells. Ketones aid healthy living and do not assist cancer cells.
2. Cancer cells spread to areas of inflammation in the body.
3. Cut cancer risk by ceasing to smoke tobacco products and reduce alcohol consumption.
4. Obesity is a potential source of cancer.
5. Some causes of cancer – chronic inflammation in the body, stress, loneliness and social isolation, bereavement, chronic depression, lack of quality sleep, electromagnetic radiation,
6. Avoid all trans fats.
7. Lower intake of processed carbohydrate foods.
8. Insulin grows cancer, Ketones and oxygen assist in the destruction of cancer cells.
9. Fasting may be beneficial in fighting cancer. Cancer cells require energy and nutrients. Fasting deprives cancer cells of these nutrients, it slows the growth of some tumours and appears to increase P53 (anti-cancer) levels.
10. Fasting reduces cancer growth, especially during chemotherapy. Fasting alone may not be enough.

Try a three-to-five-day water fast during chemotherapy.
11. Increase your Omega 3 fatty intake and avoid omega 6 fatty acids from processed seed oils and fast food.
12. Consume only grass-fed meat, rather than grain fed meat products.
13. Aim for 35g of fibre daily in your diet.
14. Eat natural antioxidant foods rather than cheap synthetic supplements.
15. Some cancer reducing foods – flax seeds, avocado, garlic, beans, lentils, cabbage, bean sprouts, berries, grapes, non-GMO soy, pumpkin and their seeds, carrots, oily fish, all nuts (avoid peanuts), unprocessed whole foods, plant-based foods, citrus fruits, and green tea.
16. A Keto food plan lowers glucose, efficiently burns ketones, and lowers insulin. Aim for a glucose/ketone ratio of 1 to 1. A keto food plan is anti-inflammatory for your body.
17. Black tea lowers carbohydrate absorption and balances post meal sugar spikes. Drink with cinnamon after your meal.
18. Lavendar and rosemary essential oils help to lower cortisol in the body by triggering GABA, the relaxation brain chemical.

Looking after Diabetic health.

Ways to improve your health if you have Type 2 Diabetes.

1. There are many options for overcoming diabetes without medication. Technically speaking, while the condition can be reversed, it cannot currently be cured. You can remove your risk for the development of diabetes complications and have consistently normal blood glucose levels, lipid

profiles and blood pressure by the following measures.
2. This repair and reversal cannot be completed by artificial means such as medication. It requires, in addition, a healthy diet filled with nutrients to conduct cellular repair. Reversal does require dietary and lifestyle maintenance to be sustained.

   Changing your diet and lifestyle are the most significant changes you can make to help reverse type 2 diabetes. It is not enough to just add exercise to your daily regime if you seek to reduce your risk of death and disease. A healthy diet and a healthy weight are imperative in the quest to change your life. Being overweight or obese is still one of the primary risk factors in the onset of type 2 diabetes.
3. The inclusion of high-fibre, low-sugar foods that are nutrient-dense but low in calories can help reduce weight and the inflammation associated with obesity. Following a healthier diet and losing weight can also reduce your blood sugar levels.

   The conventional medical food plan recommends mostly whole grains, fruits, vegetables. However, eliminating processed grains may be beneficial to patients because these grains can elicit a higher glycaemic response than other carbohydrate sources. Minimally processed foods, like sweet potatoes, may be emphasised over convenience items like bread. Some also feel that grains contain components that can be irritating and contribute to inflammation, such as gluten.
4. Fat is a necessary part of every meal to mediate the glycaemic response and slow the digestion and absorption of food, to promote slow and steady blood glucose levels. Good, wholesome fats from whole dairy products, egg yolks, fatty fish, nuts, avocados, and the like are not considered to be bad

for you.
5. Trans fats and added fats found in processed foods are what you should avoid.
6. In conventional therapy, a patient is usually recommended to consume 25 to 30 grams of fibre per day through whole grains, cereals, fruits, and vegetables. In holistic nutrition, it might be even more beneficial for patients to consume eight to ten servings of fruit and vegetables per day, so that they get the added benefits of all the phytonutrients and micronutrients found in these products.
7. In general, the holistic approach to nutrition advocates whole, natural foods as opposed to more processed foods in conjunction with a diet that is generally lower in carbohydrates, and higher in fat, protein, fibre, and micronutrients, than a conventionally prescribed diet. Several supplements in the form of vitamins, minerals and herbs have also been discovered to help alleviate the symptoms of type 2 diabetes and help bring about its reversal. It is not one vitamin or mineral or herb individually, that are able to help reverse diabetes, but rather, collectively.

It is the combination of effort on all fronts by which a person can regain their freedom from disease and reverse their diagnosis of type 2 diabetes.

Foods To Eat or Avoid for Reversing Type 2 Diabetes

Foods to Avoid

1. Sugar – Avoid. Most processed foods contain some form of added sugar for flavour enhancement, even if they don't taste sweet. All these added sugars cause extreme peaks and falls in blood glucose levels.

2. Trans Fats – totally avoid.
3. Reduced-Fat Foods - avoid since they will contain sugars to enhance flavour.
4. Processed Foods, Sugars, and Artificial Sweeteners. Processed foods are one of the biggest culprits, as it is greatly promoted by the excessive intake of added fats and sugars.
5. The sodium nitrates and nitrites found in processed meats have been found to be toxic to humans and can incite the growth of cancer cells. Nitrates and nitrites have also been linked to the onset of many diseases, including type 2 diabetes.

Foods to eat.

1. Fruits and vegetables should be the primary source of carbohydrates for a type 2 diabetic, along with whole grains. Fruits and vegetables are rich in key vitamins, minerals, and phytonutrients. This makes them very nutrient-dense choices that also happen to be low in calories (with a few exceptions).
2. Whole grains are excellent grain choices compared to bleached and processed options. Choose Whole Grains and Low-Sugar Carbohydrates. Whole grains are higher in fibre and have a much better nutrient profile.
3. Wild-Caught Fatty Fish.
4. Both lean meats that are pasture-raised and wholesome sources of plant protein like lentils should be included as part of a healthy diet for a type 2 diabetic. Some plant proteins, such as beans and legumes, also contain carbohydrates so that should be considered when planning a meal.

Key nutrients that aid in the Reversal of Type 2 Diabetes

1. Chromium - Chromium can be found in egg yolks,

nuts, green beans, broccoli, brewer's yeast, and meat.
2. Vitamin D – Your skin produces vitamin D when it's exposed to sunlight. Experts say that the skin can produce enough of the vitamin in about 30 minutes of sun exposure. This time length varies upon several factors, such as how much skin is being exposed and what time and season it is. It can be especially difficult to get enough vitamin D in the winter or if you live in a low-sunlight region. Fatty fish, such as wild salmon, trout and swordfish contain between 86 and 97% of the RDI for vitamin D per three-ounce serving. White fish and mackerel contain about 50%. Other fish such as tuna, halibut, sole and flounder are also excellent sources of vitamin D, though lower than the previous examples. Mushrooms are a great vegetarian source of vitamin D as well, with some varieties containing up to 131% of the RDI.
3. Vitamin C – Fruit and vegetables, especially oranges, strawberries, papayas, broccoli, and cauliflower.
4. Beta-Carotene – Beta-carotene, the antioxidant found in much orange and red produce that's related to vitamin A, has also been shown to fight type 2 diabetes. Consume fruits such as papaya, apricots, raspberries, cantaloupe, and watermelons and mangos. Amongst vegetables consume butternut squash, red bell peppers, carrots, summer squash, sweet potatoes, and pumpkin. Amongst green vegetables Bok choi, kale, collard greens and spinach are good sources of the nutrient as well.
5. Magnesium – In relation to diabetes, magnesium helps regulate your blood glucose. Magnesium-rich foods to include in your daily diet are leafy greens such as spinach, Swiss chard, beet, and turnip greens.

6. Seeds and nuts are another great option, including pumpkin seeds, cashews, and almonds. Also, 80% plus dark chocolate, black beans, and seafood.

Lifestyle Changes to Reverse Diabetes

1. Resistance training, such as weightlifting, and lower-intensity muscle conditioning exercises like yoga were found to be independently successful at reducing diabetes risk.
2. Tobacco - Smoking cigarettes is toxic and is associated with increased insulin resistance. This can lead to higher blood sugar levels, and the eventual development of type 2 diabetes.
3. Alcohol - Consumption of alcohol can also impede your ability to manage your blood glucose levels if you are a type 2 diabetic. Alcohol has negative effects on your liver and the way it processes fat from the blood. If you are already a diabetic, it is probably best to avoid drinking altogether.
4. Antidepressants – Antidepressants have also been associated with type 2 diabetes. A general link was found between the long-term consumption of antidepressants and an increased risk of having poor blood glucose control. Review with your healthcare professional before any decision to cease taking.
5. Being overweight is another key factor in the development of diabetes. It has also been proven by scientific studies that being overweight or obese increases the likelihood you will develop type 2 diabetes. Diabetes increases the number of years a person is likely to suffer from disability and shorten their lifespan.

Supplements to Improve Your Health

Supplements are no replacement for a healthy diet and lifestyle. They can, however, support your efforts and help assist you with reaching your goals.

1. Probiotics – Fermented vegetables, like sauerkraut, kimchi are a delicious way to eat your vegetables and get a double boost of nutritional benefits and probiotic benefits. Kefir is a popular fermented beverage that is most compared to yogurt, but it can also be made with water, grains, or coconut water. It is best to consume the unpasteurised varieties since they have a much higher probiotic content.
2. Cinnamon - One half teaspoon a day assists blood-sugar-stabilising.
3. Spirulina.
4. Chlorella.
5. Aloe Vera - Aloe vera gel can help reduce inflammation throughout the body – a common symptom of type 2 diabetes.
6. Green Tea.
7. Ginger – ginger is effective at increasing insulin sensitivity.
8. Turmeric – Researchers found that curcumin, the anti-inflammatory antioxidant compound in turmeric, may be protective against insulin resistance and type 2 diabetes by lessening the inflammatory response promoted by obesity.
9. Astaxanthin – Astaxanthin is another type of antioxidant produced by algae, yeast and sea life that has anti-inflammatory properties and a vast array of other health benefits.
10. Fish Oil – Fish oil supplementation helps control blood glucose metabolism and aids in the metabolism of fat cells.
11. Silymarin – Silymarin is an antioxidant-filled extract of milk thistle. Milk thistle has been shown

12. Chia Seeds – Contain nutrients and antioxidants that can help reverse type 2 diabetes.
   13. Magnesium – Magnesium citrate is an excellent option because it is affordable, readily available, and easily absorbed.

Conclusion - To overcome a disease like diabetes, you must also embark on a path to wellness. Health and wellness are not created by any one activity, supplement, or food: it is created through a combination of all these. So, eat clean, wholesome foods that are nutrient-dense and free of nutritionally depleted additives and ingredients. Soon, you won't crave the junk food anymore, and you may even find that you don't even like it anymore. The next step is working on your lifestyle. Exercise is key, but don't feel defeated if it's hard at first. Everything is hard when you first start out, and everything gets easier over time. Even if you just start with ten or fifteen minutes a day, that's a great way to begin a more active life. Eating well and engaging in physical activity are truly the corner stones of human health.

Looking after Eye Health

Maintaining optimum eye health is important for overall wellbeing. Here are ways to help keep your eyes healthy.

Steps to take to avoid damaging your eye health.

   1. Avoid smoking. Smoking increases the risk of eye diseases like macular degeneration and cataracts.
   2. Avoid excess alcohol. Excessive consumption can lead to vision problems, therefore drink in moderation.
   3. Control allergies that can irritate your eyes by avoiding triggers and using allergy medications.
   4. Avoid rubbing your eyes. Rubbing your eyes can introduce dirt and germ and lead to eye irritation.
   5. Restrict screen time on PCs, laptops, smart

phones, tablets and play station equipment. Reduce prolonged screen time and maintain an appropriate distance from the screens.
6. Take proactive control of conditions like diabetes and hypertension, which can seriously impact eye health.
7. Some eye diseases are hereditary, e.g., macular degeneration and glaucoma. Be aware of your family's eye health history.
8. Reduce risk of cataracts – prevent exposure to UV from the sun, avoid microwaves, avoid oxidation, avoid glycates, keep blood pressure at normal levels.

Steps to take enhance your eye health.

1. Regular eye exams: Schedule comprehensive eye examinations with an optometrist or ophthalmologist to detect and address any issues early.
2. Eat a balanced diet: Consume foods rich in Vitamin A, C, and E as well as antioxidants like lutein and zeaxanthin found in leafy greens, carrots, and eggs.
3. Stay hydrated: Drink 2 litres of water daily.
4. UV Protection: Wear sunglasses that block 100% of UVA and UVB rays to protect your eyes from harmful sun exposure.
5. Wear eye protection: Use safety goggles when engaged in activities that could cause eye injury.
6. Computers and human interaction: Position your computer monitor at eye level and take regular breaks to reduce eye strain. Apply a blue light filter to your PC, smart phone, tablet and play station equipment.
7. Proper lighting: Ensure adequate and evenly distributed lighting when reading or working.
8. Use lubricating eye drops: If you have dry eyes, use

preservative free artificial tears as needed.
9. Blink frequently: Blinking moistens the eyes, reducing dryness and irritation. Eye exercises: Practice some simple eye exercises to improve focus and reduce eye strain.
    a. Exercises include blinking for two minutes. This improves blood circulation.
    b. Big eyes, close eyes tightly for 5 seconds then open them wide. Repeat 10 times. This strengthens eyelid muscles, blood circulation and relaxes the eye muscles.
    c. Rub the palms of your hands until they become warm. Cover your eyes with your hands. After a minute open your eyes.
    d. Massage: With your fingers, gently press the upper eyelids for 2 seconds. Repeat 3 times. |This massage can improve circulation of your intraocular fluid.
    e. Rinse your eyes twice a day. In the morning do this with warm water and then in cold. In the evening do again though this time in reverse order.
    f. Hold your eyelids closed tight for 5 seconds then open sharply. Repeat 10 times.
    g. Slowly rotate the pupils in a circle. 4 times clockwise and then 4 times anticlockwise.
    h. Slowly move your eyes from left to right and then right to left. Repeat 6 times
    i. Follow the 20-20-20 rule: Take a 20 second break to look at something, 20 feet away, every 20 minutes when working on a computer.
10. Aim for 7 to 8 hours quality sleep nightly to refresh your eyes.
11. Stay active: Regular physical activity supports good blood circulation, including your eyes. Walk

in nature.

Maintaining eye health is an ongoing process. If you experience any changes in your vision or eye discomfort, consult with an eye care professional for guidance and treatment.

Key vitamins for the eyes

1. Vitamin A – from dairy, organ meats, cod liver oil.
2. Lutein and Zeaxanthin – from kale, greens, romaine lettuce, broccoli, peppers, egg yolks.
3. Zinc – from shellfish, pumpkin seeds, liver, squash, spinach, broccoli, sweet potato, red meat, and chicken.
4. Vitamin B1 – from Thiamine (water based) and Benfiotiamine (fat based)
5. Vitamin B2 and B3 – from nutritional yeast.
6. Bile salts – from ox bile.
7. Vitamin C – from fruit and vegetables, from fermented foods such as kimchi and sauerkraut. Avoid synthetic Vitamin C, Ascorbic Acid.
8. Vitamin E – from nuts, seeds, spinach, avocado.
9. Selenium – from Brazil nuts, wild fish, eggs.
10. NAC to lower body oxidation.

Diet issues

1. Avoid all processed foods.
2. Use quality fats, e.g., coconut oil, organic butter, ghee, extra virgin olive oil. Avoid all processed seed oils.
3. Include nuts and seeds in your food plan.

Looking after Heart health.

Your heart health is essential for living a holistic life. The good news is you can give your heart the assistance it needs to maintain tip top performance. Learn to treat your heart with care and respect and it will last you a lifetime. Optimising heart health is crucial for overall well-being.

Steps to take to avoid damaging your heart health.

1. Quit smoking: Smoking greatly increases the risk of heart disease. Seek support to quit.
2. Limit your alcohol intake: If you drink, do so in moderation (up to one drink per day for women, up to two for men).
3. Limit your consumption of processed foods: Reduce consumption of processed and fast foods.
4. Avoid prolonged periods of sitting. Take breaks and move regularly.

Steps to take to enhance your heart health.

1. Eat a heart-healthy diet: Consume fruits, vegetables, whole grains, and lean proteins.
2. Limit consumption of saturated fats, trans fats, salt, and added sugars. Eat Omega-3 fats: Include sources of omega-3 fatty acids, like fatty fish (such as wild salmon, sardines, mackerel, trout, herring anchovies, pilchards, and whitebait), in your diet.
3. Eat fibre-rich foods: Consume foods high in fibre, such as vegetables, fruit, nuts, seeds, oats, beans, and whole grains.
4. Stay hydrated: Drink 2 litres of water daily to support overall health.
5. Maintain a Healthy Weight: Achieve and maintain a healthy body weight through diet and exercise. Know your weight and your Body Mass Index numbers. This will enable you to check that you are on track here. Weigh yourself weekly to keep your 'finger on the pulse.'
6. Practice portion control: Be mindful of portion sizes to avoid overeating. Reduce plate sizes to assist you.

7. Exercise regularly: Aim for at least 150 minutes of moderate-intensity aerobic activity or 75 minutes of vigorous-intensity activity every week. Stay active. Engage in the exercises you enjoy.
8. Get sufficient sleep: Aim for 7-9 hours of quality sleep per night. Keep you your sleep and waking times regular. Use smart phone applications and/or smart watches to monitor sleep quality.
9. Manage your stress: Practice stress-reduction techniques like meditation, yoga, and deep breathing exercises. Start slowly and the benefits will build up over time.
10. Control your blood pressure: Monitor and manage high blood pressure through lifestyle changes or if needed medication as prescribed by your health care adviser. Take a blood pressure reading weekly to monitor progress.
11. Manage cholesterol levels: Keep cholesterol levels in check through diet, exercise, and medication if necessary. Be particularly aware of small particle LDL cholesterol levels, these are more likely to contribute to the development of heart disease.
12. Know your family heart health history: Be aware of your family's history of heart disease. Be mindful of factors like tobacco, alcohol, and sedentary lifestyles and how they affected your family.
13. Control your diabetes: If you have diabetes, manage it effectively to reduce heart disease risk.
14. Stay socially connected: Maintain strong social ties with family and friends, as social connections can benefit heart health.
15. Follow medical advice: Take regular check-ups: Schedule regular check-ups with your healthcare provider to monitor heart health. If you have specific heart-related conditions, follow your healthcare provider's recommendations closely, for

personalised guidance and to assess your risk factors.

Foods that help to reduce arterial plaque.

1. Extra Virgin Olive Oil
2. Bell peppers for vitamin C
3. Wild salmon, sardines, mackerel, trout, herring anchovies, pilchards, whitebait, and omega 3 fish oil
4. Garlic
5. Tomatoes
6. Nutritional yeast
7. Chia seeds – for fibre and to promote a healthy gut biome.
8. Fermented foods – kefir, kimchi, sauerkraut
9. Berries
10. Avocados
11. Leafy green vegetables
12. Krill oil
13. Green tea
14. Reduce and then eliminate all processed foods.

To help clear blood clots

Help to eliminate blood clots.

1. Consume avocados and green leafy greens.
2. Add turmeric, black pepper, ginger, and thyme to your diet.
3. Keep active by regular exercise.
4. Consume Natto.
5. Bromelain (from pineapple).
6. Organic apple cider vinegar.
7. Garlic.
8. Omega 3 fatty acids, flax seeds.
9. If you are overweight, lose weight.
10. Make sure you add enough potassium, sodium, and magnesium to your diet to ensure healthy heart

function.

Foods to help lower blood pressure.

1. Apples
2. Pumpkin seeds
3. Cayenne pepper
4. Roasted garlic
5. Tomatoes,
6. Lemon
7. Extra virgin olive oil
8. Beets

Foods to improve blood circulation

1. Garlic
2. Turmeric
3. Raw onions
4. Cayenne pepper
5. Wild salmon
6. Pomegranate
7. Cinnamon
8. Beets
9. Citrus fruits
10. Spinach and collard greens
11. Walnuts
12. Ginger
13. Tomatoes
14. Berries

Ways to lower resting heart rate.

1. Run
2. Hydration
3. Avoid nicotine.
4. Avoid caffeine.
5. If you are overweight, reduce your body weight.
6. Reduce stress levels, try meditation and yoga.

7. Check that the magnesium, potassium, and sodium levels are in the right balance.

Improving leg and feet blood flow

1. Wear compression socks
2. Stop smoking tobacco.
3. Eat nitrate rich fruit and vegetables, such as dark greens, cauliflower, broccoli, citrus fruits, pomegranates.
4. Manage Blood Pressure through regular exercise, lower sodium intake, lower stress levels, lower sugar intake.
5. Practice foot exercises – ankle pumps, hold both feet and legs against a wall for 20 minutes daily, clockwise and anticlockwise feet circles.

Some hidden causes of heart attacks

1. Lack of oxygen (Hypoxia)
2. A deficiency in levels of Vitamin B1 and Vitamin B12 can increase hypoxia.
3. Excess sugar in the diet and high LDL cholesterol
4. Adrenaline and stress leading to high blood glucose. High cortisol has a similar effect.
5. Be mindful of any fight/flight response during your day.
6. Avoid tobacco and vaping, they cause body stress.
7. Lower fructose in your diet.
8. Reduce alcohol intake.

Chiropractic Adjustment

1. Chiropractic adjustment dates back over 100 years when Daniel Palmer, a healer from Iowa found that misaligned vertebrae in our spines could significantly impact health. He believed that misaligned vertebrae could cause the nervous

system to malfunction, resulting in a myriad of different symptoms in many parts of the body.
2. These symptoms range from neck and back pain, through to more subtle problems such as lack of energy, problems with the digestive system, impaired immune health, and cardiovascular symptoms. Spinal misalignment increases sympathetic overdrive (the "revving up" of the nervous system) which is linked to palpitations and atrial fibrillation. Misaligned vertebrae can irritate the vagus nerve which may explain some cases of "vagus a-fib". If no obvious cardiac cause for a-fib can be established, it may be worth considering a spinal evaluation with a qualified chiropractor.
3. Vertebrae can become misaligned for many reasons, even dating back to birth. It's not just physical trauma that causes misalignment, nutritional deficiencies and emotional stress can cause it too. Even a slight misalignment in the vertebrae can throw the nervous system out of balance.
4. Misaligned vertebrae have been associated with a host of seemingly unrelated medical conditions including headaches, vision problems, including blurred vision, tinnitus non cardiac chest pain, high blood pressure, digestive problems, IBS, tiredness, fatigue, poor concentration, arthritis, joint pain, susceptibility to chronic viral infections, and impaired immune system.
5. Arrhythmia, tachycardia, and palpitations. High blood pressure is a condition which commonly accompanies atrial fibrillation and surprisingly this too can be caused by a misalignment of the atlas vertebrae in the top of the spinal column. This can cause an altered blood flow to the brain, sending the nervous system into overdrive which can increase blood pressure. Unfortunately, there have never

been any official studies done into chiropractic adjustment and atrial fibrillation, this might be due to the reluctance of some medical professions to embrace the practice. Nevertheless, there is a fair amount of anecdotal evidence with patients claiming that it has helped or even cured their atrial fibrillation.
6. If you have atrial fibrillation which has no apparent cause, and particularly if you have ever had any trauma to your back or neck then chiropractic adjustment may be of value to you. As with any form of alternative remedy always check with your doctor and consider the pros and cons.
7. *Serious complications are rare in the hands of a fully qualified and experienced practitioner, but they can include herniated discs and exacerbation of existing disc problems. Very rarely indeed, neck manipulation may lead to stroke. Some health insurance policies do cover the costs of chiropractic adjustment, although this might limit your choice of practitioner.*

Looking after Kidney Health

Maintaining optimum kidney health is crucial for overall well-being, as the kidneys play a vital role in filtering waste and excess fluids from the blood. Here are some key steps and factors to consider in achieving and maintaining kidney health:

Factors affecting your kidney health.

1. Obesity increases the potential risk for kidney problems.
2. Diabetes is a major risk factor for kidney disease.
3. Excess salt can raise blood pressure, which can be harmful to the kidneys.
4. Smoking can damage blood vessels, including those in the kidneys.

5. Overuse of non-prescription pain relievers like ibuprofen can harm the kidneys.
6. Some herbal supplements can harm the kidneys if taken in excess.
7. Watch out for urinary tract infections.
8. Conditions like hypertension, and kidney stones can impact your kidney health.
9. Excess phosphorus from foods in your diet can harm the kidneys.

Steps to enhance your kidney health.

1. Hydration: Drink an adequate amount of water to support kidney function. Dehydration can strain kidney function. Drink 2 litres of water daily.
2. Maintain a healthy weight through a balanced diet and regular exercise. Obesity can increase the risk of kidney problems.
3. Follow a diet that is low in processed foods and high in fruits, vegetables, whole grains, and lean proteins. This can help prevent conditions like high blood pressure and diabetes that can harm the kidneys.
4. Reduce sodium intake by avoiding high sodium processed foods.
5. Excessive alcohol consumption can strain the kidneys.
6. High blood pressure is a leading cause of kidney damage. Monitor your blood pressure on a weekly basis and work with a healthcare provider to manage it.
7. If you are diabetic, manage your blood sugar levels carefully.
8. Alcohol: Drinking in moderation is vital for kidney health.
9. Quit smoking is very beneficial for kidney health.
10. Engage in regular physical activity to support

overall health. Exercise can help control blood pressure and maintain a healthy weight.
11. Sleep: Aim for 7-8 hours of quality sleep per night to support overall health.
12. Manage Stress: Chronic stress affects your body's systems, including the kidneys. Practice stress-reduction techniques like meditation, deep breathing, or yoga.
13. Limit your use of over-the-counter pain medications. Only use as directed on the package.
14. Herbal Supplements: Avoid overuse of herbal supplements by consulting with a healthcare provider before using them.
15. Be hygiene aware: Practice good hygiene to prevent urinary tract infections (UTIs), which can affect your kidney health. Ensure proper hygiene, especially when using public conveniences, to help prevent urinary tract infections (UTIs).
16. Be proactive in managing any chronic health conditions.
17. Limit your intake of processed foods: Reduce consumption of processed and high-phosphorus foods.

Some practical tips to aid your kidney health.

1. Be mindful of oxalates, they are found in almonds, spinach, beet tops, grains, Swiss chard, turmeric, kiwi fruit and can adversely impact your kidneys.
2. Watch for malabsorption in the gut from low stomach acidity. This can lead to higher calcium levels in the blood.
3. Sugar is toxic for the kidneys.
4. If eating oxalate foods add dairy (cheese) to offset any adverse effect.
5. Citrus fruits can lower symptoms of gout and help

protect against kidney stones.
6. Organic apple cider vinegar can help reduce kidney stones.
7. Eat foods high in potassium and low in oxalates.
8. Eat micro greens – they are high in nutrients, add to salads. Micro greens have beneficial sulforaphane, chlorophyl, flavonoids and catenoids.
9. Check your electrolyte balance – the ratio of sodium, potassium, and magnesium intake.
10. Ketones are good for the kidneys.

Seek professional guidance: Consult with your healthcare provider for personalised guidance and to assess your specific risk factors. Schedule regular check-ups to monitor your kidney function through blood and urine tests. Also discuss the latest research and recommendations regarding kidney health.

Small, consistent lifestyle changes can have a significant impact on kidney health. By adopting the holistic approach and you can tailor your strategies to your individual needs and circumstances.

Looking after Liver health.

The liver plays several vital functions in the body, including:
1. The liver helps to metabolise nutrients from food, converting them into energy, storing glucose as glycogen, and processing fats and proteins.
2. The liver detoxifies harmful substances, such as drugs and alcohol, by breaking them down into less toxic forms.
3. The liver produces bile, essential for digestion. Bile helps emulsify fats, making it easier for the body to absorb them.
4. The liver stores essential nutrients like vitamins, minerals, and glycogen for later use by the body.
5. The liver regulates blood composition, including

filtering toxins and waste products, and producing proteins necessary for blood clotting.
6. The liver plays a role in the immune system by removing bacteria and other foreign particles from the blood.

Thus, the liver is a crucial organ that performs multiple functions vital for maintaining overall health and well-being.

Some of the best ways to maintain a healthy liver:

1. Eat a balanced diet rich in fruits, vegetables, whole grains, lean protein, and healthy fats. Limit or eliminate your intake of processed foods, sugar, and saturated fats.
2. Drinking an adequate amount of water helps your liver function properly and flush out toxins. Consume 2 litres daily.
3. Be moderate in in your alcohol consumption. The Chief Medical Officers advice for men and women is that it is safest to drink no more than 14 units of alcohol per week. This should be spread over 3 or more days in that week. In between, there should be several alcohol-free days. Above all avoid binge drinking.
4. Engage in regular physical activity to help maintain a healthy weight and reduce the risk of fatty liver disease.
5. Being overweight can contribute to liver problems. Being overweight, with the concentration visible around the solar plexus can indicate the onset of fatty liver disease. To reverse this, achieve and maintain a healthy weight through diet and exercise.
6. Practice safe sex and never sharing needles. Hepatitis B and C can be transmitted through unprotected sex and needle sharing.

Take precautions to prevent these infections. Vaccinations are available for hepatitis A and B. Consider getting vaccinated if you're at risk.
7. Only take medications and supplements as prescribed or recommended by a healthcare professional, as some are hard on the liver.
8. Wash your hands regularly to prevent the spread of infections that can affect the liver.
9. If you have conditions like diabetes, high blood pressure, or high cholesterol, work with your healthcare provider to manage them effectively.
10. Limit your exposure to environmental toxins and chemicals that can harm the liver.
11. Moderate caffeine intake is generally safe, excessive caffeine and sugary beverages can contribute to liver issues. Consume them only in moderation.
12. Visit your healthcare provider for routine check-ups and liver function tests to detect any issues early.

If you have concerns about your liver or specific health conditions, consult a healthcare professional for personalised guidance.

Foods to promote a healthy liver.

1. Increase fibre with fruit and vegetables. Such as Apples, Avocados, Parsley, Beetroot, Leafy green vegetables
2. Green Tea
3. Garlic
4. Up your vitamin C from citrus fruits and fermented foods
5. Turmeric
6. Nuts
7. Extra virgin olive oil

Helpful liver nutrients

1. Choline from leafy greens

2. Methionine from eggs, Brazil nuts
3. Sulforaphane from leafy green vegetables and vegetable sprouts

Signs of fatty liver disease

1. Right hand shoulder pain, from blocked or clogged bile ducts
2. Large pot shaped belly
3. Severe rib pain on your right-hand side
4. Spider veins from excess oestrogen
5. Man boobs.
6. Swollen right foot (Oedema) from poor circulation. Itchy palms and on the soles of the feet
7. Hypothyroidism
8. Constant fatigue from low vitamin absorption (Affecting vitamins A, D, E and K)

Some ways to reverse fatty liver.

1. Cut out all inflammatory vegetable seeds oils.
2. Avoid processed grains and caffeine.
3. Eliminate sugar and starchy carbohydrates from your diet.
4. Stop snacking between main meals, try intermittent fasting.
5. Take a quality digestive enzyme (Bile salts, pancreatin, Betain Hydrochloride).
6. Choline
7. Eat Sulphur rich vegetables (such as garlic, asparagus, onions, leeks).
8. Eat cruciferous vegetables.
9. Consider taking Milk Thistle and Glutathione.
10. Drink lemon water.
11. Drink organic apple cider vinegar.
12. Ginger – helps lower fatty liver and lowers LDL cholesterol while increasing HDL cholesterol and

lowers body inflammation.
13. Take Tudca for liver health, this helps with the bile issue. Tudca helps boost bile flow from the liver. Tudca helps to lower glutamate toxicity, protects mitochondria, and enhances energy levels. Good for gut biome and lowers gut inflammation, protects brain function, and may reduce insulin resistance.
14. Eat bitter sour foods artichokes, dark greens. Eat fermented foods, sauerkraut, kimchi, and kefir. Eat raw foods, organ meats and wild fish.

Ways to enhance liver function.

1. With your GP review your medications and if advised reduce.
2. Lower intake of sugar and starchy carbohydrates.
3. Lower Fructose consumption.
4. Avoid cooked canned foods, alcohol, junk food, corn (low vitamin content).
5. Avoid processed vegetable seed oils,
6. Avoid whey protein powder.
7. Avoid Maltodextrin (synthetic glucose)
8. Avoid Alfa Toxins in peanuts and corn.
9. Monosodium Glutamate (MSG, a fast-food flavour enhancer.)
10. Be conscious of Isolates in food, they can affect liver function.
11. Avoid Soy protein isolates.

Looking after Prostate Health

Here are ways to optimise prostate health.
1. Limit the consumption of red meat and processed foods.
2. Don't smoke or quit if you currently do.

3. Limit alcohol consumption.
4. Limit the use of over-the-counter decongestants and antihistamines.
5. Avoid prolonged sitting or standing when possible.
6. Maintain a balanced diet rich in fruits and vegetables.
7. Eat foods high in antioxidants, such as tomatoes and berries.
8. Stay hydrated by drinking plenty of water.
9. The key vitamins for prostate health are Zinc, Vitamin C and Vitamin D.
10. Engage in regular physical activity and exercise.
11. Pelvic floor exercises, like Kegels, can help with prostate health.
12. Maintain a healthy body weight.
13. Manage stress through relaxation techniques or meditation.
14. Practice safe sex to reduce the risk of sexually transmitted infections.
15. Ensure regular and healthy bowel movements to reduce pressure on the prostate.
16. Consider herbal supplements or medications under the guidance of a healthcare professional if necessary.
17. Know your family history of prostate issues.
18. Be aware of potential prostate cancer symptoms, such as urinary changes or pain.
19. Discuss prostate health with your doctor, especially after age 50. Consider prostate-specific antigen (PSA) testing if recommended by your doctor.

Remember that it's essential to consult with a healthcare provider for personalised advice and screenings related to prostate health, as individual circumstances can vary.

GERARD ANTHONY LANKESTER

Mastering Holistic Wellness,
A Practical Guide for Every Day.

CHAPTER 5 - THE MIND

Managing Emotions

Fostering positive thought patterns and cultivating empowering self-talk are powerful tools for personal growth and well-being. Here are ways to achieve this:

1. Recognise negative thought patterns: Begin by developing awareness of negative thought patterns that may be holding you back. Pay attention to the self-limiting beliefs and negative self-talk that arise in your mind. Recognising these patterns is the first step towards transforming them. Unhappy people blame the outer world. Happy people build their inner world.
2. Challenge negative thoughts: Once you become aware of negative thoughts, challenge them with rational and positive perspectives. Ask yourself if there is evidence to support these negative beliefs or if they are based on assumptions or past experiences. Replace negative thoughts with more realistic and positive affirmations. It is important to acknowledge that conviction is more powerful than positive thinking. Conviction guides you through misfortune, it does not wish it away. Conviction and purpose outdo positivity.
3. Practice self-compassion: Treat yourself with kindness and compassion. Replace self-criticism with self-acceptance and self-love. When faced with

setbacks or challenges, remind yourself that you are doing your best and that mistakes are opportunities for growth. Cultivating self-compassion helps shift your mindset towards positivity and resilience.

4. Affirmations and positive self-talk: Use affirmations and positive self-talk to rewire your thinking patterns. Create a list of empowering statements that resonate with you and repeat them daily. For example, affirmations like "I am capable of achieving my goals" or "I embrace challenges as opportunities for growth" can help shift your mindset towards optimism and self-belief.

5. Surround yourself with positivity: Surround yourself with positive influences and supportive people. Choose relationships, environments, and media that uplift and inspire you. Engage in activities that bring you joy and fulfilment. The more you immerse yourself in positivity, the easier it becomes to maintain positive thought patterns and self-talk.

6. Gratitude practice: Cultivate a gratitude practice to foster a positive mindset. Each day, take a moment to reflect on and appreciate the things you are grateful for. This practice helps shift your focus towards the positive aspects of your life, enhancing your overall well-being.

7. Visualisation and goal setting: Utilise visualisation techniques to envision your desired outcomes and goals. Create a clear mental image of what you want to achieve and use positive self-talk to reinforce your belief in your abilities. Visualising success and speaking positively about your goals helps manifest them into reality.

8. Mindful thought monitoring: Practice mindfulness to observe your thoughts without judgment. When negative or self-limiting thoughts arise,

gently redirect your focus to more positive and empowering thoughts. Mindfulness allows you to detach from negative thought patterns and choose more supportive ways of thinking.
9. (Ralph Waldo Emerson) "For every minute you are angry, you lose sixty seconds of happiness."
10. Personal development and learning: Engage in personal development activities and continuous learning. Reading self-help books, attending workshops, or listening to podcasts that focus on personal growth can provide you with tools and insights to foster positive thought patterns and develop empowering self-talk.

Fostering positive thought patterns and cultivating empowering self-talk is a journey that requires consistent practice and self-awareness. By applying these practical strategies in your daily life, you can rewire your thinking, boost self-confidence, and create a more positive and empowering mindset.

Applying practical techniques to foster positive thought patterns and cultivate empowering self-talk in your day-to-day life can have a profound impact on your overall well-being.

Practical ways to implement these techniques:

1. Daily affirmations: Start your day by repeating positive affirmations that resonate with you. Choose empowering statements such as "I am capable and deserving of success," "I embrace challenges as opportunities for growth," or "I have the power to create positive change." Repeat these affirmations throughout the day, especially when you encounter self-doubt or negative thoughts.
2. Thought awareness: Develop a habit of being aware of your thoughts. Pay attention to the narratives

playing in your mind and notice when negative or self-limiting thoughts arise. This awareness is the first step towards challenging and transforming them into positive and empowering ones.

3. If you are depressed, you are living in the past; if you are anxious, you are living in the future; at peace, you are living in the present.
4. Reframing: Practice reframing negative thoughts into more positive and constructive perspectives. When you catch yourself engaging in negative self-talk, consciously reframe it by finding alternative, empowering interpretations. For example, instead of thinking, "I always mess things up," reframe it as, "I am learning and growing from my experiences."
5. Gratitude practice: Incorporate a daily gratitude practice into your routine. Take a few minutes each day to reflect on and express gratitude for the positive aspects of your life. This practice helps shift your focus from what's wrong to what's right, fostering a positive mindset and empowering self-talk.
6. Surround yourself with positivity: Surround yourself with positive influences, whether it's supportive friends, uplifting books, inspiring podcasts, or motivational quotes. Create a positive environment that nurtures and reinforces empowering self-talk. Limit exposure to negative news or toxic relationships that can trigger self-doubt or negativity.
7. Self-Compassion: Practice self-compassion by treating yourself with kindness and understanding. Be gentle with yourself when faced with challenges or setbacks. Replace self-criticism with self-encouragement and self-acceptance. Treat yourself as you would a dear friend, offering words of support and understanding.

8. Mindfulness meditation: Incorporate mindfulness meditation into your daily routine. Set aside a few minutes each day to focus on your breath, observe your thoughts without judgment, and bring your attention back to the present moment. This practice cultivates a sense of calm, helps you detach from negative thought patterns, and promotes self-awareness.
9. Journaling: Keep a journal to capture your thoughts, emotions, and experiences. Use it as a tool for self-reflection and self-discovery. Write down positive affirmations, record moments of gratitude, and challenge negative thoughts by finding evidence to the contrary. Journaling allows you to gain insights into your thinking patterns and helps redirect them towards positivity.
10. Seek support: Surround yourself with a supportive network of family, friends, or a mentor who can provide encouragement and accountability. Share your goals and aspirations with them and seek their guidance and support in fostering positive thought patterns and empowering self-talk.
11. Continuous learning: Engage in personal development activities that promote continuous learning and growth. Read self-help books, attend workshops, or listen to podcasts that focus on positive psychology, personal growth, and mindset. Expand your knowledge and adopt new tools and techniques to further enhance your positive thought patterns and self-talk.

By consistently applying these practical techniques in your day-to-day life, you can foster positive thought patterns and cultivate empowering self-talk. It takes time and practice to rewire your thinking, but with dedication and persistence, you can create a mindset that supports your well-being and helps you achieve your goals.

Managing Stress

Managing stress effectively is crucial for maintaining optimal well-being. When left unaddressed, chronic stress can negatively impact both your physical and mental health.
'If you can make improvements to your body, you can do the same for your mind.'

Key strategies to manage stress and understand its impact on your overall well-being

1. Identify Stress Triggers: Start by identifying the specific factors that contribute to your stress. Recognise the situations, events, or even thoughts that tend to generate stress responses. This self-awareness will help you better understand and manage your stress levels.
2. Practice stress reduction techniques: Explore various stress reduction techniques and find what works best for you. This could include deep breathing exercises, mindfulness meditation, progressive muscle relaxation, or engaging in hobbies and activities that bring you joy. Experiment with different techniques and incorporate them into your daily routine to alleviate stress.
3. Prioritise Self-Care: Make self-care a priority in your life. Ensure you are getting enough restful sleep, maintaining a balanced diet, and engaging in regular physical activity. Taking care of your physical and mental health strengthens your resilience to stress and helps you cope better with life's challenges. Dedicate time each day for self-care activities that help you relax and recharge.

This could include reading, taking a warm bath, practicing yoga or meditation, or engaging in a hobby you enjoy. Making self-care a non-negotiable part of your day it helps to your reduce stress and promotes a sense of well-being.

4. Cultivate supportive relationships: Surround yourself with a supportive network of family, friends, or professionals who can provide emotional support and guidance. Sharing your feelings and concerns with others can help lighten the load and provide valuable perspective and advice. Sharing your feelings and experiences with trusted individuals can provide comfort, advice, and a sense of connection. Surrounding yourself with a supportive network helps alleviate stress and promotes emotional well-being.

5. Time management and boundaries: Effectively manage your time and establish boundaries to prevent overwhelm and burnout. Learn to prioritise tasks, delegate responsibilities when possible, and say no to additional commitments when necessary. Setting clear boundaries helps protect your well-being and reduce unnecessary stress. Efficiently managing your time can alleviate stress. Prioritise tasks and create a realistic schedule, allowing for breaks and downtime. Break larger tasks into smaller, manageable steps, and tackle them one at a time. By organising your time effectively, you can reduce personal overwhelm and increase productivity.

6. Practice mindfulness: Incorporate mindfulness into your daily life by staying present and fully engaged in the present moment. Pay attention to your thoughts, emotions, and physical sensations without judgment. Mindfulness allows you to detach from stressful thoughts and cultivate a sense

of calm and clarity.
7. Seek professional help: If stress becomes overwhelming or affects your daily functioning, consider seeking professional help. Therapists, counsellors, or coaches can provide guidance, tools, and support to help you manage stress effectively.

Understanding the impact of stress on your overall well-being is crucial. Chronic stress can lead to a range of health problems, including cardiovascular issues, weakened immune system, anxiety, and depression. By managing stress effectively, you reduce these risks and promote better physical, mental, and emotional health.

Remember, everyone's stress triggers and coping mechanisms differ. Take the time to understand yourself and experiment with different strategies until you find what works best for you. With consistent practice and a proactive approach to stress management, you can lead a more balanced and fulfilling life. Implementing strategies to manage stress effectively on a day-to-day basis is essential for maintaining your overall well-being.

Practical ways to incorporate stress management techniques into your daily routine

1. Practice deep breathing: Throughout the day, take moments to focus on your breath. Practice deep breathing exercises by taking slow, deep breaths in through your nose and exhaling through your mouth. Deep breathing triggers the relaxation response and calms the nervous system, reducing stress levels.
2. Take regular breaks: Incorporate regular breaks into your schedule to give yourself a mental and physical pause. Step away from your work or daily tasks and engage in a brief relaxation practice, such as stretching, walking outdoors, or listening to

calming music. These breaks help rejuvenate your mind and prevent burnout.
3. Engage in physical activity: Physical activity is a powerful stress reliever. Find time for regular exercise, whether it's a brisk walk, a workout session at the gym, or participating in a sport you enjoy. Exercise releases endorphins, improves mood, and helps reduce stress hormones in the body.
4. Establish healthy boundaries: Know your boundaries and set boundaries in both your personal and professional life. Say, 'No' to excessive commitments that may cause stress and learn to delegate tasks when possible. Setting boundaries helps prevent overwhelm and ensures you have time for self-care and relaxation.
5. Connect with nature: Spending time in nature has a calming effect on the mind and body. Take short walks in green spaces, spend time in your garden, or simply sit outside and soak in the natural surroundings. Connecting with nature helps reduce stress, enhances mood, and promotes overall well-being.
6. Practice gratitude: Cultivate a gratitude practice by reflecting on the positive aspects of your life. Each day, take a moment to identify things you are grateful for and write them down. Focusing on gratitude helps shift your perspective, reduces stress, and fosters a positive mindset.

Managing stress is a lifelong practice, and what works for one person may not work for another. Explore different techniques, be patient with yourself, and adapt your stress management strategies as needed. Incorporating these day-to-day practices, you can build resilience, reduce stress levels, and cultivate a greater sense of balance and well-being in your life.

Developing Mindfulness

Developing mindfulness practices can be immensely helpful in reducing anxiety and increasing mental clarity.

Practical ways to incorporate mindfulness into your daily routine:

1. Start with mindful breathing: Take a few moments each day to focus on your breath. Sit or lie down in a comfortable position, close your eyes, and bring your attention to your breath. Notice the sensation of each inhale and exhale, letting go of any thoughts or distractions that arise. This simple practice can help calm your mind and reduce anxiety.
2. Engage in mindful activities: Infuse mindfulness into your everyday activities by bringing full awareness to the present moment. Whether you're eating, walking, or doing household chores, pay attention to the sensations, smells, tastes, and movements involved. Engaging in activities mindfully helps to anchor your attention to the present and cultivates a sense of calm.
3. Practice body scan meditation: Set aside a few minutes each day for a body scan meditation. Lie down or sit in a comfortable position and slowly direct your attention to each part of your body, starting from your toes and moving up to your head. Notice any sensations, tensions, or areas of relaxation without judgment. This practice promotes self-awareness and relaxation.
4. Develop an attitude of gratitude and appreciation: Take time to reflect on the things you appreciate in your life. Write down three things you're grateful for each day, whether big or small. This practice shifts your focus towards positivity and helps to

reduce anxiety by fostering a sense of contentment and perspective.
5. Practice mindful eating: Pay attention to your eating habits and approach meals with mindfulness. Slow down, savour each bite, and observe the flavours, textures, and smells of the food. Develop the habit of chewing your food 20 times before swallowing.
6. Incorporate mindful movement: Engage in mindful movement practices such as yoga, tai chi, or qigong. These practices combine gentle physical movements with breath awareness and promote relaxation, stress reduction, and improved mental clarity.
7. Embrace mindful listening: When engaging in conversations or interactions with others, practice mindful listening. Give your full attention to the person speaking, truly hear their words, and avoid interrupting or formulating responses in your mind. Mindful listening fosters deeper connections and improves understanding.
8. Create mindful transitions: Introduce mindfulness into transitions between tasks or activities. Before moving from one task to another, take a moment to pause, centre yourself, and set your intention for the next activity. This practice helps to bring focus and clarity to each new endeavour.
9. Practice Loving-Kindness meditation: Dedicate time to loving-kindness meditation, where you extend well-wishes and compassion to yourself and others. Cultivating a sense of kindness and empathy reduces anxiety and fosters a positive mindset.

Incorporating these mindfulness practices will enable you, with time, to reduce anxiety, enhance mental clarity, and cultivate a greater sense of peace and well-being. Mindfulness is a skill that develops with regular practice and patience. Embrace the present moment, nurture self-compassion, and allow mindfulness to become an integral part of your journey towards holistic wellness. Developing mindfulness and meditation practices and incorporating them into your day-to-day life can be a transformative journey towards reducing anxiety and increasing mental clarity.

Meditation is gym for the mind.

1. Initially set aside time to sit in a quiet space, focus on your breath, and bring your attention to the present moment.
2. Meditation, what is it? It can be structured and formal, equally it can be informal and be just as valid. Some examples - taking a walk-in nature, taking a hike, listening to the birds. Notice wherever and whenever a sense of ease arises, and the mind becomes calm. Be aware of these moments through your day when you naturally experience a meditative state. It is something you will uncover from within.
3. The peace that you seek is not 'peace of mind' but 'peace from mind.'
4. You have 2 choices with your mind, control your mind or let your mind control you. The purpose of meditation is not to control your thoughts, it is to stop letting your thoughts control you.
5. Transform your perception of distractions when meditating, learn to use any distraction (e.g., pain, focus on your pain). The more difficult the distraction, the better it is.
6. See your thoughts and emotions as like clouds in the sky, fleeting and ever changing. See you mind as the sky, stable and ever there. So, always treat your thoughts as passing experiences. They do not define who you are.

Practical ways to apply these techniques:

1. Morning mindfulness meditation ritual: Begin your day with a few minutes of mindfulness practice. Starting your day with mindfulness meditation sets a positive tone and helps cultivate a calm and focused mindset.
2. Mindful check-ins: Throughout the day, take mindful pauses to check in with yourself to notice how you are feeling emotionally, mentally, and physically. Allow yourself to acknowledge and accept any emotions or sensations without judgment. This practice helps you stay connected with yourself and identify any areas of anxiety or stress that may arise.
3. Mindful breathing: Incorporate mindful breathing exercises into your daily routine. Whenever you feel overwhelmed or anxious, take a few deep breaths, focusing on the sensation of the breath entering and leaving your body. This simple practice helps calm the nervous system and brings you back to the present moment. Slow down your breathing by counting to 4 on the in breath, and count to 6 on the out breath. Such a practice will slow your breathing rate to 6 or 7 breaths per minute and will increase your body's supply of oxygen to the lungs.
4. Mindful observation: Engage in mindful observation exercises to cultivate present-moment awareness. Take a few minutes each day to observe your surroundings with curiosity and without judgment. Notice the colours, shapes, textures, and sounds around you. This practice enhances your ability to be fully present and reduces anxiety by shifting your focus away from racing thoughts.
5. Mindful walking: During your daily walks or when moving from one place to another, practice mindful walking. Pay attention to the sensations of your feet

touching the ground, the movement of your body, and the sounds in your environment. This form of moving meditation helps ground you in the present moment and increases your overall sense of well-being.

6. Mindful eating: Bring mindfulness to your meals by savouring each bite and fully engaging your senses. Take time to appreciate the colours, flavours, and textures of your food. Chew slowly and be present with each mouthful. This practice not only enhances your enjoyment of food but also supports better digestion and reduces stress-related eating. In addition, it enhances your enjoyment and creates a deeper connection with the nourishment you provide your body.

7. Mindful exercising - Engage in mindful movement practices such as yoga, tai chi, or qigong. These practices combine gentle physical movements with breath awareness and promote relaxation, stress reduction, and improved mental clarity.

8. Mindful listening - When engaging in conversations or interactions with others, practice mindful listening. Give your full attention to the person speaking, truly hear their words, and avoid interrupting or formulating responses in your mind. Mindful listening fosters deeper connections and improves understanding.

9. Mindful technology usage: Practice mindfulness while using technology by setting boundaries and being intentional. Avoid multitasking and bring your full attention to one task at a time. Limit unnecessary screen time and create technology-free zones or periods during your day. Being mindful of your technology use helps reduce digital distractions and promotes mental clarity.

10. Mindful Self-Care: Engage in activities that nourish

your mind, body, and soul. Whether it's taking a warm bath, practicing yoga, reading a book, or engaging in a creative hobby, approach these activities with mindfulness. Fully immerse yourself in the present moment, savouring the experience and allowing it to rejuvenate you.

11. Evening reflection: Dedicate a few minutes each evening to reflect on your day. Practice gratitude by acknowledging the positive moments and expressing appreciation for them. Also, reflect on any challenging moments with self-compassion and seek to learn lessons and growth opportunities. This reflection cultivates a sense of balance and helps ease anxiety before bedtime.

12. Bedtime mindfulness: End your day with a bedtime mindfulness practice to promote restful sleep. Engage in relaxation techniques, such as progressive muscle relaxation or guided meditation, to calm your mind and release tension from your body. Focus on your breath and allow any thoughts or worries to gently drift away. Reflect on your day and if any matters need action on the following day, note these thoughts on a pad. By writing down these thoughts you release them from your mind.

Recognising and managing your emotions effectively is a crucial aspect of holistic wellness.

1. Emotional awareness – Start by developing a deeper understanding of your emotions. Pay attention to how you feel in different situations and identify the specific emotions you experience. Becoming aware of your emotions is the first step in managing them effectively. (Epictetus) "It isn't events that disturb people, rather their mind judgements about them."

All events are inanimate and objective. The is little purpose in getting angry or sad about things that are indifferent to our feelings.
2. Mindfulness practice – Cultivate a regular mindfulness practice to enhance your emotional awareness. Mindfulness involves being fully present in the moment and non-judgmentally observing your thoughts and emotions. Through mindfulness, you can develop a greater sense of self-awareness and gain insight into the triggers and patterns behind your emotional experiences.
3. Emotional regulation techniques - Learn practical techniques to regulate your emotions when they become overwhelming. Deep breathing exercises, progressive muscle relaxation, and visualisation are examples of effective techniques that can help you calm your mind and body in stressful or emotional situations.
4. Self-Reflection and journaling - Take time for self-reflection and introspection to better understand the underlying causes of your emotions. Consider keeping a journal where you can write about your emotions, their triggers, and any patterns you notice. This process can help you gain clarity and insight into your emotional responses.
5. Healthy coping mechanisms - Engage in healthy coping mechanisms to manage and express your emotions constructively. Engaging in physical activity, pursuing creative outlets, practicing mindfulness, or seeking support from loved ones are all healthy ways to channel and process your emotions. Avoid harmful coping mechanisms such as substance abuse or excessive indulgence in unhealthy behaviours.
6. Emotional Intelligence - Cultivate emotional intelligence, which involves understanding and

managing your own emotions while also empathising with the emotions of others. Developing empathy and practicing active listening can enhance your interpersonal relationships and lead to healthier emotional dynamics.

7. Seek support - Don't hesitate to seek support from trusted friends, family members, or professionals when needed. Talking about your emotions with a supportive listener can provide valuable insights and help you navigate challenging emotions more effectively. Therapists or counsellors can offer guidance and teach you additional strategies for managing your emotions.

8. Self-Care - Prioritise self-care to support your emotional well-being. Engage in activities that bring you joy, relaxation, and rejuvenation. Take care of your physical health through exercise, proper nutrition, and adequate sleep, as these factors can significantly influence your emotional state.

9. Mindful communication - Practice mindful communication to express your emotions effectively and assertively. Choose to actively listen to others and express yourself in a respectful and constructive manner. Effective communication can foster healthier relationships and prevent emotional conflicts.

10. Continuous growth - Embrace personal growth as an ongoing journey. Recognise that managing emotions is a skill that can be developed over time. Stay open to learning, seek self-improvement resources, and be patient with yourself as you navigate your emotional landscape.

By recognising and managing your emotions effectively, you can experience greater emotional well-being, improved relationships, and enhanced overall holistic wellness.

Remember, it takes practice and self-compassion to develop these skills, so be gentle with yourself throughout the process.

Some practical ways to manage your emotions.

1. Emotional check-ins - Set aside a few moments each day for an emotional check-in. Take a few deep breaths and ask yourself how you're feeling. Notice any emotions that arise without judgment or criticism. This practice helps you develop a habit of tuning into your emotional state regularly.
2. Emotional journaling - Keep an emotions journal where you can record your daily experiences and the corresponding emotions. Reflect on the situations or triggers that evoke strong emotions in you. This practice allows you to identify patterns and gain insights into the underlying causes of your emotions.
3. Name your emotions - Practice labelling your emotions by giving them names. When you experience a specific emotion, consciously identify it by saying, "I am feeling [emotion]." This simple act of naming helps create distance between you and the emotion, allowing you to observe it more objectively.
4. Releasing your emotions - In a fight/flight situation, once through it, it is imperative to release the emotional energy from your body. So, scream, shout, shake your body stamp your feet, until all the toxic emotional energy from your body has gone. This is practiced throughout the animal kingdom, only humans have placed social constraints on releasing emotional energy. Retaining these false social constraints in your life is toxic for your body.
5. Pause and reflect - Develop the habit of pausing before reacting to strong emotions. When you

encounter a challenging or triggering situation, take a moment to step back and reflect. Consider the possible consequences of your immediate reactions and choose a response that aligns with your values and promotes emotional well-being.

6. Practice emotional acceptance - Instead of suppressing or avoiding difficult emotions, practice accepting them as a natural part of being human. Allow yourself to fully experience and acknowledge your emotions without judgment. Embracing your emotions with acceptance reduces their intensity and creates space for growth and healing.

7. Emotional regulation techniques - Learn and practice specific techniques for regulating your emotions in real-time. Deep breathing exercises, grounding techniques, or mindfulness meditation can help calm your nervous system and bring you back to a state of balance. Experiment with different techniques to find what works best for you.

   When considering an emotional situation apply the following - Those things within your sphere of control, act on. Those emotional situations outside of your control, ignore.

8. Develop empathy - Cultivate empathy towards yourself and others. Practice putting yourself in someone else's shoes to better understand their emotions. This empathetic perspective fosters compassion and helps you respond to emotions, both yours and others', with greater understanding and kindness.

9. Self-Care - Prioritise self-care activities that nurture your emotional well-being. Engage in activities that bring you joy, relaxation, and comfort. This may include taking walks in nature, practicing hobbies you enjoy, spending quality time with loved ones, or engaging in creative outlets.

10. Continuous Learning - Embrace learning opportunities to deepen your understanding of emotions and emotional intelligence. Read books, attend workshops, or listen to podcasts on emotional well-being and self-awareness. Continuous learning expands your emotional vocabulary and equips you with practical tools to navigate and manage your emotions effectively.
11. Seek support: - Reach out to a trusted friend, family member, or therapist when you need support in managing your emotions. Talking about your emotions with a supportive listener can provide validation, guidance, and fresh perspectives on how to navigate challenging emotional situations.

By incorporating these practical day-to-day strategies, you can cultivate emotional intelligence, develop greater self-awareness, and manage your emotions more effectively. Remember, it's a process that requires patience, self-compassion, and consistent practice. Over time, you'll develop resilience and emotional well-being that positively impacts all areas of your life.

How to build emotional resilience and coping mechanisms for navigating life's challenges.

1. Understand resilience - Begin by understanding what resilience means and how it applies to your emotional well-being. Resilience is the ability to bounce back from adversity, adapt to change, and maintain a positive outlook. Recognise that resilience is a skill that can be developed and strengthened over time.
2. Identify personal strengths - Reflect on your personal strengths and qualities that have helped you overcome difficult situations in the past. Recognising your inner resources and resilience can

boost your confidence and provide a foundation for developing effective coping mechanisms.
3. Positive Self-Talk - Practice positive self-talk to cultivate a resilient mindset. Challenge negative or self-defeating thoughts and replace them with positive and empowering affirmations. Remind yourself of your strengths, past successes, and your ability to handle challenges.
4. Seek social support - Build a strong support network of friends, family, or support groups who can provide emotional support during challenging times. Reach out to trusted individuals who can listen, offer guidance, and provide a fresh perspective on your situation. Connecting with others can help you feel understood, validated, and strengthen your resilience.
5. Develop coping mechanisms - Explore and develop healthy coping mechanisms that work for you. Engage in activities that help you relax, reduce stress, and process emotions effectively. This may include exercise, journaling, engaging in hobbies, practicing mindfulness or meditation, or seeking therapy. Experiment with different strategies to find what resonates with you.
6. Embrace change and adaptability - Life is full of changes, and cultivating a mindset of adaptability can enhance your resilience. Embrace change as an opportunity for growth, learn from setbacks, and approach challenges with a flexible and open mindset. Recognise that change can lead to new possibilities and personal development.
7. Practice Self-Care: Prioritise self-care to nurture your emotional well-being and build resilience. Ensure you are getting enough restful sleep, maintaining a balanced diet, and engaging in activities that bring you joy and relaxation. Taking

care of your physical and emotional needs equips you to better cope with stress and adversity.
8. Cultivate emotional intelligence - Develop your emotional intelligence to understand and manage your emotions effectively. This involves being aware of your emotions, recognising their triggers, and responding to them in a healthy and constructive manner. By cultivating emotional intelligence, you can navigate challenges with greater emotional resilience.
9. Learn from adversity - View adversity as an opportunity for growth and learning. Reflect on past challenges and identify the lessons you've gained from those experiences. Use those insights to develop a more resilient mindset and prepare yourself for future obstacles.
10. Foster optimism - Cultivate optimism by focusing on the positive aspects of your life, nurturing gratitude, and practicing optimism even during challenging times. Optimism enhances resilience by helping you maintain a positive outlook, find silver linings, and approach difficulties with hope and perseverance.
11. Prioritise quality time - Set aside dedicated time each day to spend with your loved ones. It could be having a meal together, going for a walk, or engaging in an activity that you both enjoy. Focus on being fully present, actively listening, and engaging in meaningful conversations to deepen your emotional connection.
12. Practice Active Listening - When engaging in conversations, make a conscious effort to practice active listening. Give your full attention, maintain eye contact, and show genuine interest in what the other person is saying. Avoid distractions and refrain from interrupting. By truly listening,

you validate the other person's feelings and perspectives, fostering a deeper connection.
13. Express appreciation and gratitude - Take a moment each day to express appreciation and gratitude to the important people in your life. Be specific in acknowledging their positive qualities, actions, or support. Genuine expressions of gratitude strengthen bonds and create a positive atmosphere in relationships.
14. Show empathy and understanding - Practice empathy by putting yourself in the other person's shoes. Seek to understand their emotions and perspectives without judgment. Show compassion and validate their feelings. This fosters a sense of emotional safety and deepens the connection between you and the other person.
15. Engage in meaningful conversations - Initiate meaningful conversations that go beyond surface-level topics. Ask open-ended questions, encourage the other person to share their thoughts and feelings, and actively participate in the discussion. Sharing vulnerabilities and engaging in deeper conversations nurtures emotional connections.
16. Practice random acts of kindness - Surprise your loved ones with small acts of kindness and thoughtfulness. It could be leaving a heartfelt note, preparing their favourite meal, or helping with a task. These acts of kindness show that you care and strengthen the emotional bond between you and the other person.
17. Practice forgiveness and letting go - Cultivate forgiveness and let go of past resentments or grudges. Holding onto negative emotions hinders emotional connections. Practice forgiveness by having open and honest conversations, expressing your feelings, and working towards reconciliation.

Letting go allows for growth and deepens the emotional connection.
18. Support each other's dreams and goals - Encourage and support the aspirations and goals of your loved ones. Celebrate their achievements and aid when needed by being a source of support and encouragement, you build a foundation of trust and strengthen the emotional connection.
19. Practice nonjudgmental acceptance - Embrace the uniqueness of each individual and practice nonjudgmental acceptance. Allow others to express themselves authentically without fear of criticism or rejection. Accepting others for who they are fosters a deep sense of connection and strengthens relationships.
20. Engage in shared activities - Engage in activities that you both enjoy and that create shared experiences. It could be participating in a hobby, going on adventures, or pursuing a common interest. Shared activities create memories and deepen the emotional bond between you and the other person.

By incorporating these practical day-to-day ways into your life, you can enhance your relationships and foster deeper emotional connections. It takes effort, patience, and genuine care to build strong and meaningful connections, but the rewards are invaluable for your holistic well-being and the well-being of those around you.

Developing Positive Thought Patterns - Foster positive thought patterns and cultivate empowering self-talk using the following.

1. Recognise negative thought patterns - Begin by developing awareness of negative thought patterns

that may be holding you back. Pay attention to the self-limiting beliefs and negative self-talk that arise in your mind. Pay attention to the narratives playing in your mind and notice when negative or self-limiting thoughts arise. This awareness is the first step towards challenging and transforming them into positive and empowering ones.
2. Challenge negative thoughts - Once you become aware of negative thoughts, challenge them with rational and positive alternatives. Ask yourself if there is evidence to support these negative beliefs or if they are based on assumptions or past experiences. Replace negative thoughts with more realistic and positive affirmations. Start your day by repeating positive affirmations that resonate with you. Choose empowering statements such as "I am capable and deserving of success," or "I have the power to create positive change." Repeat these affirmations throughout the day, especially when you encounter self-doubt or negative thoughts.
3. Practice self-compassion: Treat yourself with kindness and compassion. Replace self-criticism with self-acceptance and self-love. When faced with setbacks or challenges, remind yourself that you are doing your best and that mistakes are opportunities for growth. Cultivating self-compassion helps shift your mindset towards positivity and resilience.
  (Christopher Germer) "Self-compassion is simply giving the same kindness to yourself that you would give to others."
4. Affirmations and positive self-talk - Use affirmations to rewire your thinking patterns. Create a list of empowering statements that resonate with you and repeat them daily. For example, an affirmation like "I embrace challenges as opportunities for personal growth," can help

shift your mindset towards self-belief. So, instead of thinking, "I always mess things up," reframe the thought as, "I am learning and growing from my experiences."

5. Surround yourself with positivity - Surround yourself with positive influences and supportive people. Choose relationships, environments, and media that uplift and inspire you. Engage in activities that bring you joy and fulfilment. Surround yourself with positive influences, whether it's supportive friends, uplifting books, inspiring podcasts, or motivational quotes. Create a positive environment that nurtures and reinforces empowering self-talk. Limit exposure to negative news or toxic relationships that can trigger self-doubt or negativity. The more you immerse yourself in positivity, the easier it becomes to maintain your positive outlook on life.

6. Gratitude practice - Cultivate a gratitude practice to foster a positive mindset. Each day, take a moment to reflect on and appreciate at least 3 things you are grateful for. This practice helps shift your focus towards the positive aspects of your life, enhancing your overall well-being.

7. Visualisation and goal setting - Utilise visualisation techniques to envision your desired outcomes and goals. Create a clear mental image of what you want to achieve, this will reinforce your belief in your abilities. Visualising success and speaking positively about your goals helps to bring them into reality.

8. Mindful thought monitoring - Practice mindfulness to observe your thoughts without judgment. When negative or self-limiting thoughts arise, gently redirect your focus to more positive and empowering thoughts. Set aside a few minutes each day to focus on your breath, observe your thoughts

without judgment, and bring your attention back to the present moment. This practice cultivates a sense of calm, helps you detach from negative thought patterns, and promotes self-awareness.
9. Personal development and learning - Engage in personal development activities and continuous learning. Reading self-help books, attending workshops, or listening to podcasts that focus on personal growth can provide you with tools and insights. Expand your knowledge and adopt new tools and techniques to further enhance your positive thought patterns and self-talk.
10. Journaling - Keep a journal to capture your thoughts, emotions, and experiences. Use it as a tool for self-reflection and self-discovery. Write down positive affirmations, record moments of gratitude, and challenge negative thoughts by finding evidence to the contrary. Journaling allows you to gain insights into your thinking patterns and helps redirect them towards positivity.
11. Seek Support - Surround yourself with a supportive network of family, friends, or a mentor who can provide encouragement and accountability. Share your goals and aspirations with them and seek their guidance and support in fostering positive thought patterns and empowering self-talk.

Fostering positive thought patterns and cultivating empowering self-talk is a lifelong journey that requires consistent practice. Applying these practical strategies in your daily life, you rewire your thinking, boost your self-confidence, and create a more positive and empowering mindset.

How to sharpen mental focus.

Learning techniques to sharpen mental focus and concentration is essential for enhancing productivity, improving cognitive performance, and achieving success in various areas of life.

Practical ways to sharpen your mental focus and bring into your daily routine:

1. Practice mindfulness meditation - Engage in regular mindfulness meditation sessions to train your mind to stay focused on the present moment. Sit in a quiet space, close your eyes, and bring your attention to your breath. Whenever your mind wanders, gently redirect your focus back to the breath. Over time, this practice strengthens your ability to concentrate and reduces distractions.

2. Meditation is akin to taking out all your furniture, home contents, and placing them outside. You then decide what to bring back inside and what to dispose of. All this is conducted through the act of conscious breathing.

3. Set clear goals and prioritise tasks - Clearly define your goals and break them down into smaller, manageable tasks. Prioritise your tasks based on importance and urgency and create a structured plan for tackling them. By having a clear direction, you can eliminate mental clutter and stay focused on the task at hand.

4. Create a distraction-free environment - Minimise distractions in your environment to optimise your focus. Find a quiet space, free from unnecessary noise or interruptions. Silence your phone, close unnecessary tabs on your computer, and create a clutter-free workspace. A clean and organised environment promotes mental clarity and enhances concentration.

5. Utilise time blocking techniques - Time blocking involves allocating specific time periods for dedicated tasks or activities. Set aside uninterrupted

blocks of time for focused work and resist the temptation to multitask. By allocating dedicated time slots for specific tasks, you can maintain sustained focus and accomplish more in less time.

6. Practice single tasking - Instead of multitasking, focus on one task at a time. Multitasking divides your attention and reduces productivity. Give your full attention to each task, complete it, and then move on to the next. This approach improves concentration and allows for deeper engagement with each activity.

7. Take regular mental breaks - Breaks are crucial for maintaining mental focus and preventing mental fatigue. Incorporate short breaks into your schedule to recharge your mind. Engage in activities that relax and rejuvenate you, such as stretching, deep breathing exercises, or going for a brief walk. These breaks replenish your mental energy and enhance your ability to concentrate.

8. Exercise regularly - Physical exercise not only benefits your body but also enhances mental focus. Engaging in regular exercise increases blood flow to the brain, promotes the release of mood-boosting endorphins, and improves cognitive function. Incorporate aerobic exercises, such as brisk walking, jogging, or cycling, into your routine to sharpen mental focus.

9. Practice mindful eating - Nourish your brain with a balanced and nutritious diet. Choose foods that support brain health, such as fruits, vegetables, whole grains, and healthy fats. Practice mindful eating by savouring each bite, paying attention to the flavours and textures of your food. Proper nutrition provides the fuel your brain needs to stay focused and sharp.

10. Get sufficient sleep - Quality sleep is crucial

for optimal cognitive function and concentration. Prioritise getting enough sleep each night to allow your brain to rest and recharge. Establish a consistent sleep routine and create a relaxing environment conducive to sleep. Quality sleep enhances mental clarity, attention, and focus.

Applying practical ways of to sharpen your mental focus and on a day-to-day basis.

1. Start with mindful morning rituals - Begin your day with a mindful morning routine to set a focused tone for the rest of the day. Engage in activities such as meditation, journaling, or light stretching to centre your mind and enhance mental clarity.
2. Break tasks into smaller chunks - large tasks can be overwhelming and lead to a lack of focus. Break them down into smaller, more manageable chunks. By tackling one task at a time, you can maintain concentration and experience a sense of accomplishment along the way.
3. Use time-management techniques - Implement time-management techniques such as the Pomodoro Technique. Set a timer for a specific work interval, typically 25 minutes, and fully immerse yourself in the task at hand. Take a short break, around 5 minutes, between each interval to recharge your focus.
4. Minimise distractions - Consider using website blockers or apps that limit distractions during focused work periods.
5. Practice active listening: - When engaging in conversations or attending meetings, practice active listening. Give your full attention to the speaker,

maintain eye contact, and ask clarifying questions. This helps improve your focus on the conversation and enhances your understanding of the topic.

6. Incorporate regular movement breaks - Physical movement is linked to improved cognitive function. Take short movement breaks throughout the day to stretch, go for a short walk, or do some light exercises. Physical activity boosts blood flow to the brain, helping to enhance focus and concentration.

7. Stay hydrated and nourished - Dehydration and poor nutrition can negatively impact cognitive function. Drink plenty of water throughout the day to stay hydrated, as even mild dehydration can affect focus. Fuel your body with balanced meals that include brain-boosting foods like fruits, vegetables, whole grains, and lean proteins.

8. Practice mindful technology use - Limit your exposure to excessive screen time and practice mindful technology use. Set specific times for checking emails and social media and avoid mindless scrolling. Designate technology-free periods during your day to cultivate uninterrupted focus.

9. Take regular mental breaks - Allow yourself short mental breaks to prevent mental fatigue and maintain focus. Engage in activities that relax your mind, such as deep breathing exercises, meditation, or listening to calming music. These breaks provide a reset for your brain and improve your ability to concentrate.

10. Prioritise quality sleep - Getting sufficient sleep is vital for optimal cognitive function. Establish a consistent sleep schedule and create a sleep-friendly environment. Practice good sleep hygiene by avoiding stimulating activities before bed and creating a relaxing bedtime routine.

Applying these practical techniques to your day-to-day life, can sharpen your mental focus and concentration, leading to increased productivity and improved cognitive performance. Consistency and practice are key to developing and maintaining these skills. With time, you'll notice a significant enhancement in your ability to achieve this.

Reflections on the Mind

Setting boundaries - how you can get your life back

1. Set personal boundaries, of your own beliefs and be conscious of the beliefs. Be aware of the ways that keep you from knowing how to respect yourself. Not setting boundaries can stem from fear. (Fear of loss or rejection)
2. Be mindful that there is no guarantee that people will meet you on your terms. Just be sufficiently confident to say, "I respect myself enough to remove myself from this dynamic."
3. Never forget, boundaries empower you.

Your morning routine for a great life

1. Sleep, aim for seven to eight hours daily.
2. On getting up, make your bed. Show pride in your personal space.
3. Exercise in the morning.
4. Take a one-minute cold shower daily.
5. Morning meditation.
6. Set a new goal to achieve every day.
7. Be aware of what you say 'Yes' and 'No' to each day.
8. Have a schedule for your day.
9. Do challenging things which gratify you later in the day, week, month, year.
10. Have a daily routine which you follow. Do not miss

two or three days in a row because discipline is essential. But also remember you are human and not flawless.
11. Be thankful for another day of life.

At the end of every day before sleep

1. Congratulate yourself on what went well.
2. Identify problems, learn from them, and rectify.
3. Record on pen and paper, anything that is carrying over to the future.
4. Ask the question, 'how have your life goals moved forward today?'

Things to let go of

1. Failed and toxic relationships.
2. Be conscious of negatives you feed your mind; replace with positives.
3. Jealousy.
4. Past failures, regrets, misfortunes, unachieved goals.
5. Judgements of others, other people's opinions.
6. Expectations of being happy all the time.
7. Perfectionism, fear of failure, catastrophic thinking.
8. Needing to convince others that you are right.

Things to give up if you seek happiness.

1. Complaining
2. Limiting beliefs
3. Blaming others
4. Negative self-talk
5. Dwelling on the past
6. Resistance fuels suffering. Change is part of life, accept rather than resisting it. Change is never painful, only the resistance to change.
7. The need to impress others.

8. The need to be right.
9. The need for the approval of others.
10. (Bruce Lee) "Don't speak negatively about yourself, even as a joke. The body does not know the difference, words are energy and cast spells, that is why it is called spelling. Change the way you speak about yourself and change your life. What you are not changing you are also choosing."

Traits of mentally tough people

1. Able to disentangle from things they cannot influence.
2. Flexible in handling events.
3. Strong self-awareness.
4. Face up to uncertain circumstance. (Von Moltke) "No battle plan survives contact with the enemy."
5. Bounces back from disappointments.
6. Able to regulate negativity and move forward with purpose.
7. Practical optimism. Seeing opportunities where the world only sees disaster and hopelessness. (Winston Churchill) "The positive thinker sees the invisible, feels the intangible, and achieves the impossible."

Ways to enhance self-discipline.

1. Create a tension free and clutter free environment.
2. Create an action plan.
3. Take consistent small steps forward.
4. Commit to doing nothing but the task in hand.
5. Delay gratification and grow accustomed to short term setbacks.

Increase your mental strength.

1. Take 10 to 15 minutes daily and self-reflect.
2. Practice meditation regularly.

3. Focus on your purpose. Identify your challenges and set goals.
4. Ignore all things outside and beyond your personal control.
5. Replace your inner critic with your inner optimist.
6. Guard your physical health.
7. Ask yourself, "What is the worst thing that can happen?"
8. Venture beyond your comfort zone. (Robin Sharma) "The more time you spend in your discomfort zone, the more your comfort zone will expand."
9. Become comfortable with risk taking. Do one tough thing every day. Give up one bad habit every month.

Know your strengths and weaknesses.

1. Keep a gratitude journal.
2. Master new skills. Write down five new ideas daily, build your ideas muscle.
3. Live in and create a healthy environment at home and at work.

Things you control.

1. Your attitude.
2. Your thoughts.
3. People you surround yourself with.
4. Your wellbeing.
5. How you treat others.
6. Whether you ask for help or not.
7. Gratitude for what you have.
8. How you spend and invest your money.
9. Whether you try again after a setback.
10. Your daily habits.

To be emotionally healthy

1. Work on being difficult to take offence.

2. Make things fun whenever possible.
3. Do not judge others, just be curious and interested in understanding why people do what they do and say what they say.
4. Emotionally healthy people know what their needs, wants, and preferences are. They are comfortable sharing in a kind and caring way.

(Albert Camus) 'Have a motivation for living. Do not fit in, be yourself, always. Live intensively for your biggest goals. Live like a rebel. Focus on practical things. Accept the unpredictability of life. Find happiness in every phase of life because life carries you towards death.'

Mastering Holistic Wellness,
A Practical Guide for Every Day.

CHAPTER 6 - THE SPIRIT

Embracing Spiritual Growth

Exploring the role of spirituality in holistic wellness opens a path to deeper self-discovery, purpose, and inner peace. Spirituality is a personal journey that encompasses the connection to something greater than oneself and the exploration of meaning and purpose in life. It goes beyond religious beliefs and rituals, encompassing a broader sense of connection to the world, others, and oneself. Integrating spirituality into your holistic wellness journey can bring profound benefits to your overall well-being.

Key aspects to consider.

1. Connection to Self: Spirituality invites self-reflection and introspection. It encourages you to delve into your core values, beliefs, and desires. Take time for self-exploration through practices such as meditation, journaling, or mindful contemplation. Connect with your inner self, listening to your intuition, and aligning your actions with your authentic values.
2. Meaning and Purpose: Exploring spirituality involves seeking meaning and purpose in life. Reflect on what truly matters to you, what brings you joy, and what gives your life a sense of purpose. Engage in activities that align with your values and contribute to a greater good. This brings a deep sense of fulfilment and enhances your overall well-

being.
3. Connection to Nature: Embrace the beauty and interconnectedness of the natural world. Spend time in nature, whether it's taking walks in the park, hiking in the mountains, or simply appreciating a garden. Recognise the profound wisdom and healing power of nature, allowing it to nourish your mind, body, and spirit.
4. Mindfulness and Presence: Cultivate mindfulness by practicing present-moment awareness. Be fully engaged in the here and now, savouring the present experience without judgment or attachment. Engage in mindfulness practices such as mindful breathing, body scans, or sensory awareness to deepen your spiritual connection and promote a sense of calm and clarity.
5. Rituals and Sacred Practices: Explore rituals and sacred practices that resonate with you. These can include prayer, meditation, chanting, or engaging in specific rituals that hold personal significance. Rituals provide a sense of grounding, connection, and reverence, helping you tap into a deeper spiritual dimension.
6. Compassion and Service: Embrace the value of compassion and service to others. Engage in acts of kindness, volunteer work, or supporting causes that are meaningful to you. By extending compassion and contributing to the well-being of others, you nurture your own spiritual growth and foster a sense of interconnectedness.
7. Seeking Wisdom and Knowledge: Engage in the exploration of spiritual wisdom and knowledge through reading, attending workshops or seminars, or seeking guidance from spiritual mentors or teachers. Explore various philosophical and spiritual traditions, integrating what resonates with you into your own unique spiritual journey.
8. Remember, spirituality is a deeply personal and individual experience. Embrace the aspects that align with your values and beliefs and allow yourself the freedom to evolve and adapt on your

spiritual path. By exploring the role of spirituality in holistic wellness, you open the door to a profound sense of connection, purpose, and inner peace.

Exploring the role of spirituality in holistic wellness is a journey that can be incorporated into your day-to-day life in practical and meaningful ways.

Some practical suggestions for applying these techniques:

1. Morning Reflection: Start your day with a few moments of reflection or meditation. Set aside a few minutes each morning to connect with your inner self, express gratitude for the day ahead, and set positive intentions. Connecting with nature, take a few moments to step outside and breathe in the fresh air. Greet the sun, listen to the birds singing, and appreciate the beauty of the natural world around you. Then set an intention for the day, aligning yourself with the energy and wisdom of nature.
2. Mindful Practices: Infuse mindfulness into your daily activities. Whether you're eating, walking, or engaging in routine tasks, bring your full awareness to the present moment. Notice the sensations, thoughts, and emotions that arise without judgment. This practice allows you to deepen your connection to the present and cultivate a sense of spirituality in everyday life.
3. Nature Connection: Spend time in nature regularly to nourish your spiritual connection. Take walks in parks, gardens, or natural areas. Observe the beauty around you, listen to the sounds of nature, and appreciate the interconnectedness of all living beings. Allow yourself to be present in nature, finding solace, inspiration, and a sense of connection to something greater.
4. Mindful Nature Observation: Practice mindful observation when in nature. Take a few moments to be fully present and notice the intricate details of plants, the movement of animals, or the rhythm of natural elements. Engage all your senses, from

the scent of flowers to the feel of the earth beneath your feet. This mindful connection allows you to experience a deeper sense of connection and appreciate the beauty and wisdom of the natural world.
5. Nature Rituals: Create rituals that honour your connection to nature. This can be as simple as a daily gratitude practice, where you express appreciation for the gifts of nature in your life. You can also create rituals around specific natural phenomena, such as watching the sunrise or sunset, offering thanks for the changing seasons, or participating in ceremonial practices that celebrate nature's cycles.
6. Gardening and Plant Care: Engage in gardening or plant care to cultivate a deeper bond with nature. Whether you have a small indoor plant or a backyard garden, tending to plants allows you to connect with the life force and cycles of growth and renewal. As you nurture plants, you also nurture your own sense of well-being and spiritual connection.
7. Nature-Based Practices: Explore nature-based practices such as forest bathing, nature meditation, or nature-inspired art. These practices invite you to immerse yourself in nature's healing energies and tap into your own innate wisdom and creativity. They offer an opportunity to deepen your spiritual connection and experience a profound sense of peace and harmony.
8. Nature Journaling: Keep a nature journal to document your experiences and reflections in nature. Spend a few minutes each day observing and writing about the natural world around you. Describe the sights, sounds, and feelings you encounter. Capture moments of awe, gratitude, and insights that arise from your connection with nature. This practice deepens your awareness and strengthens your bond with the environment.
9. Outdoor Meditation: Find a quiet spot in nature where you can sit or lie down comfortably. Close your eyes and focus on your breath, allowing

yourself to become deeply attuned to the natural rhythm of the surroundings. Let go of thoughts and distractions, and simply be present in the moment. This meditation practice helps you cultivate a sense of unity with nature and fosters a deep sense of peace and connection.

10. Cultivate gratitude for the gifts of nature. Each day, take a moment to reflect on and appreciate the wonders of the environment. Express gratitude for the sun, the rain, the trees, and all the elements that sustain life. This practice shifts your focus to the abundance and interconnectedness of nature, fostering a deep sense of gratitude and reverence.

11. Nature-Based Creativity: Engage in creative activities inspired by nature. Paint, draw, or photograph the beauty around you. Write poems or stories inspired by the natural elements. Create nature-inspired crafts or sculptures. Engaging in artistic expressions that are rooted in nature allows you to tap into your creative flow and deepen your connection with the natural world.

12. Environmental Stewardship: Embrace your role as an environmental steward. Take actions that support the well-being of the planet, such as reducing waste, conserving resources, or participating in local environmental initiatives. By caring for the environment, you not only contribute to the greater good but also deepen your spiritual connection and sense of responsibility.

13. Retreats and Nature Immersions: Consider participating in retreats or nature immersions to deepen your connection with nature. These experiences provide an opportunity to unplug from the demands of daily life, immerse yourself in the beauty of natural surroundings, and engage in spiritual practices that foster a profound sense of connection and rejuvenation.

14. Sacred Spaces: Create a sacred space in your home where you can engage in spiritual practices. This space can be a corner with a meditation cushion, candles, crystals, or objects that hold personal

meaning. Dedicate time each day to sit quietly in this space, engage in prayer, meditation, or simply reflect on your spiritual journey.
15. Rituals and Ceremonies: Incorporate rituals and ceremonies into your life to honour your spiritual beliefs. This can include lighting candles, saying affirmations, performing gratitude rituals, or engaging in personal rituals that hold significance for you. These rituals provide a sense of sacredness, deepen your connection to spirituality, and bring mindfulness to your actions.
16. Seek Inspiration: Surround yourself with sources of spiritual inspiration. Read books, listen to podcasts, or watch videos that explore spirituality, mindfulness, and personal growth. Engage in discussions with like-minded individuals or join spiritual communities online or in person. Seek out teachers, mentors, or guides who can provide wisdom and support on your spiritual journey.
17. Gratitude Practice: Set aside dedicated time for gratitude meditation. Find a comfortable position, close your eyes, and recall the things you are grateful for. As you focus on each item, allow the feeling of gratitude to fill your heart and radiate throughout your body. This meditation practice enhances your sense of well-being and trains your mind to naturally gravitate towards gratitude.
18. Journaling and Self-Reflection: Dedicate time for journaling and self-reflection. Write about your spiritual experiences, insights, and observations. Reflect on the positive aspects of your life, big or small, and express your appreciation. This practice shifts your focus to the blessings and abundance that surround you, fostering a sense of gratitude and opening your heart to the present moment.
19. Mindful Eating: Slow down and savour each bite of your meals. Engage your senses fully as you eat, paying attention to the flavours, textures, and aromas. Be present in the experience of nourishing your body. Express gratitude for the food on your plate, the farmers who grew it, and the hands that

prepared it. This mindful eating practice brings awareness to the nourishment you receive and deepens your connection to the act of eating.
20. Acts of Kindness: Infuse your daily life with acts of kindness and compassion. Seek opportunities to help others, show empathy, and practice random acts of kindness. Offer a helping hand, lend an ear, or perform small acts of generosity. Engaging in selfless acts cultivates a sense of connection, gratitude, and spiritual fulfilment.

Spirituality is deeply personal, and there is no right or wrong way to explore it. Allow yourself the freedom to experiment with different practices and approaches and find what resonates with you. Allow nature to be your teacher, guide, and source of inspiration. As you nurture your spiritual well-being through this connection, you will find greater harmony, peace, and a deep sense of belonging to the web of life.

Cultivating gratitude and mindfulness

1. Morning Gratitude Ritual: Begin your day by expressing gratitude for the blessings in your life. Take a few moments each morning to reflect on the things you are thankful for. It could be the people you love, your health, a comfortable home, or opportunities that lie ahead. Write them down in a gratitude journal or simply say them out loud. This practice sets a positive tone for the day and helps you focus on the abundance in your life.
2. Mindful Moments: Incorporate mindfulness into your daily routines. Whether it's brushing your teeth, having a cup of tea, or taking a shower, bring your full attention to the present moment. Notice the sensations, sounds, and scents around you. Let go of distractions and simply be present with your experience. This cultivates a sense of mindfulness and helps you appreciate the simple joys of everyday life.
3. Gratitude Reminders: Place visual cues or reminders

in your environment to prompt gratitude throughout the day. It could be sticky notes with gratitude quotes on your mirror, a gratitude stone on your desk, or a gratitude app on your phone. These reminders serve as gentle prompts to pause, reflect, and express gratitude during your busy schedule.
4. Gratitude for Others: Take time each day to express gratitude towards others. Write a thank-you note, send a heartfelt message, or simply tell someone how much you appreciate them. Cultivating gratitude towards others strengthens relationships, spreads positivity, and deepens your own sense of gratitude.
5. Gratitude in Challenging Times: Train yourself to find gratitude even in difficult situations. When facing challenges or setbacks, ask yourself, "What lessons can I learn from this? What opportunities might arise?" Shifting your perspective to find the silver linings in tough times helps cultivate resilience and gratitude for growth.
6. Evening Reflection: Before bed, take a few minutes to reflect on the day and identify three things you are grateful for. It could be moments of joy, achievements, acts of kindness, or lessons learned. This reflection allows you to end the day on a positive note and fosters a sense of gratitude and contentment.

Cultivating gratitude and mindfulness is a journey, and it takes consistent practice. You will, over time, experience increased happiness, reduced stress, and a deeper appreciation for the beauty and abundance in each moment.

Journaling

Set aside regular time for journaling to reflect on your thoughts, emotions, and experiences. Write freely without judgment, allowing your thoughts to flow onto the pages. Explore your dreams, goals, challenges, and successes. This practice helps you gain insights, uncover patterns, and identify areas for personal growth.

1. Mindful Self-Reflection: Carve out moments of stillness and solitude for self-reflection. Find a quiet space where you can sit comfortably and focus your attention inward. Observe your thoughts, emotions, and physical sensations without attachment or judgment. This practice cultivates self-awareness, allowing you to better understand yourself and make conscious choices.
2. Seeking Feedback: Actively seek feedback from trusted individuals in your life. Ask for honest assessments of your strengths, areas for improvement, and blind spots. This feedback provides valuable perspectives and insights that can support your personal growth journey.
3. Learning and Personal Development: Engage in continuous learning and personal development. Read books, attend workshops or seminars, enrol in online courses, or listen to podcasts that align with your interests and goals. Acquiring new knowledge and skills expands your perspectives, fosters personal growth, and opens doors to new possibilities.
4. Goal Setting: Set meaningful and achievable goals for personal growth. Break them down into smaller, actionable steps and create a plan to work towards them. Regularly review your progress, celebrate milestones, and adjust your goals as needed. This process keeps you focused, motivated, and committed to your personal growth journey.
5. Embracing Challenges and Growth Opportunities: Embrace challenges as opportunities for growth. Instead of shying away from discomfort, lean into it with curiosity and openness. Challenge yourself to step outside your comfort zone, try new experiences, and embrace unfamiliar situations. Each challenge presents an opportunity for self-reflection, learning, and personal growth.
6. Cultivating Self-Compassion: Practice self-compassion by treating yourself with kindness, understanding, and acceptance. Embrace your

imperfections, acknowledge your efforts, and be gentle with yourself during difficult times. Self-compassion creates a nurturing environment for personal growth, allowing you to learn from mistakes and bounce back stronger.
7. Seeking Guidance and Support: Don't hesitate to seek guidance from mentors, coaches, or therapists who can provide objective perspectives, tools, and strategies to support your personal growth. They can help you navigate challenges, explore new perspectives, and unlock your full potential.

Engaging in practices for self-reflection and personal growth empowers you to live a more intentional and fulfilling life. It helps you develop a deeper understanding of yourself, uncover your passions and purpose, and navigate life's challenges with resilience and authenticity.

Reflections on the Spirit

On spiritual connectedness - Remember, with every breath you inhale 26 sextillion molecules of air. Allow it to connect with all the people in your life. Everyone you know is also breathing air that once you inhaled. Also, your breath connects with all who came before you. It might also include molecules your ancestors once breathed. You are also likely to be breathing molecules of air once inhaled and exhaled by people from all over the world. Some of the air molecules you inhaled may have been also inhaled by some of the great figures in history down the ages. Be inspired by these thoughts, feel awe at the big picture and feel the interconnection.

Stoic steps

1. Meditate.
2. See your life as though from a view high above to garner perspective.
3. Consider negative visualisation in so doing there are then no surprises.
4. Live with the contemplation of a sage.
5. Be aware of your character throughout the day.

6. Love and accept all that happens to you.
7. Separate the self from your emotions.
8. In dealing with others show compassion and understanding.
9. Grow your muscle of discipline.
10. Impermanence is part of life so simply accept.
11. Review your day every day.
12. Rest, relax and let go.

Stoic productivity strategy

1. Excellence is a habit.
2. Ask yourself the question, "Is this essential?"
3. Tackle the difficult first.
4. Focus on the small wins.
5. Say 'No' a lot.

The Self

1. In life, you play out two possibilities, from fear (limitation, contraction, and skepticism) or from love (expansion, openness, and possibility). Choose!
2. Only blame holds you back from a healed and self-empowered life.
3. No emotion is bad, it is simply telling us a story.
4. Philosophy calls for simple living, but not for penance. Hold yourself to a higher standard, but not an impossible one.
5. Hope and fear are both projections into the future, both are enemies of the present moment.
6. Know the difference between healthy self-enquiry and rumination. Rumination dwells on a problem, the negative and does not seek a solution.
7. (Anurag Ray) "Be thankful to all those people who have hurt you or disappointed you because they are the ones who made you wise and strong."
8. Never be prisoner of your past. It was just a lesson, not a life sentence.
9. (Jim Hightower) "The opposite of courage is not cowardice, it is conformity. Even a dead fish can go with the flow."

10. When fear is on top, that is the body talking. When love is on top, that is the soul guiding. Surrender your every fear, see only love. You should enjoy the brief time you have on earth and not be enslaved to emotions that make you miserable and dissatisfied.

The Self – Positive

1. View every challenge as an opportunity to exercise your virtue.
2. Choose your company well, choose those who extol virtue and cultivate their character.
3. Speak without judging. Are you aware of all the facts, if not, how can you judge a situation fairly?
4. Live life from your authentic self, that is from within.
5. Your character is not defined by what you say, rather by what you do.
6. Be tolerant of others and strict with yourself.
7. Your boundaries are your self-rules that prevent others from using you. Know what you will and will not accept. Create boundaries that honour these things, then stand by them, unquestioningly.
8. A reflection - the past is unalterable, the present is transitory, the future is uncertain. So, live your life through activities meaningful to your own life vision.
9. Happiness is a habit.
10. To achieve your dreams, embrace change, embrace risk and hard work with a winning mindset and some luck. Above all never give up.
11. Quiet the mind and the soul will speak.
12. In life better to be a seeker than a believer. A seeker is open to possibilities. A believer has found the answer and may be closed to new ideas.
13. (Amish proverb) Instead of putting others in their place, put yourself in their place.
14. Look at others' accomplishments and think, "if they can do it, why can't I?" See the success of others as a source of inspiration.

15. Before sleep reconnect with your day's activities, reconnect to a greater sense of life's meaning.

Life

1. You are a soul residing in a body. Let your soul direct your actions in all things, never the other way round.
2. Time - value it always, it is limited. Don't prepare, live it now. Life is short, don't fritter it away on non-essential obligations.
3. You will only have one shot at today. Will you fully inhabit all this day, before it slips through your fingers, and it becomes the past?
4. The Buddhist way - right intent, right speech, right action, right livelihood, right effort, right mindfulness, right concentration.
5. Take time to replenish your spirit, it allows you to serve others from the overflow. You cannot serve from an empty vessel.
6. To guarantee a good day, do good things.
7. (Nelson Mandela) "I never lose, either I win, or I learn."
8. Mistakes help you to learn and grow. Without mistakes you remain static. No one is perfect, so practice forgiving yourself.
9. (Winston Churchill) "Success is stumbling from failure to failure with no loss of enthusiasm."
10. See every challenge as an opportunity to gain insight and meaning in life.
11. Create meaning and purpose by training your mind to feel a greater sense of purpose. Forget the minutiae and focus on the truly important.
12. Inner qualities such as virtue, justice, honesty, discipline, and courage are the only things, and so worth striving for.
13. (Marcus Aurelius) "It is essential to remember that

the attention you give to any action should be in due proportion to its worth."
14. Success is no accident, it is made up of hard work, perseverance, study, and sacrifice.
15. (Karl Jung) "Who looks outside, dreams, who looks inside, awakes."
16. The work of living is to set standards and live up to them.
17. The universe is in continuous change, your understanding of what something is, is merely a snapshot.
18. See not the adult, but the child within, who was born innocent and pure, just like you.
19. Leave your mark by embodying your values and making them visible to others. That will leave a real impact and effect the world.
20. Never regret a day of your life. Good days give you happiness. Bad days give you experience. Worst days give you lessons. The best days give you memories.
21. Apply the 10,000-hour rule. Regardless of aptitude, mastery takes 10,000 hours of focused intention and practice. Thus, the seed of greatness exists in every human being. Whether it sprouts or not is your choice, great talent is nothing more than unwavering dedication to a process. The other factor is opportunities; opportunities are more like a whisper than a foghorn.
22. (Lou Redmond) "Make your definition of success something you can achieve this week rather than in ten years. Have a long-term goal but also give yourself the opportunity to be successful now." Ask yourself, how can I be successful today?
23. On becoming the best at what you do - Value creativity over comfort. Value knowledge over attention. Value intuition over conventional. Value

joyful over security. Value alive time over dead time.

(Sam Altman) *"Extreme people get extreme results. You cannot be normal and expect abnormal results."*

Mastering Holistic Wellness,
A Practical Guide for Every Day.

CHAPTER 7 - INTEGRATING HOLISTIC WELLNESS INTO YOUR DAILY LIFE.

General principles

Creating a personalised holistic wellness plan that suits your lifestyle is key to achieving long-lasting well-being. Here are some ideas on how to develop such a plan:

1. Assess Your Current Lifestyle: Begin by evaluating your current lifestyle and identifying areas that require improvement. Reflect on your daily routines, habits, and practices related to nutrition, exercise, sleep, stress management, and self-care. Take note of both positive and negative aspects, as this will guide you in building a more balanced and fulfilling wellness plan.
2. Prioritise Self-Care: Make self-care a non-negotiable part of your daily routine. Dedicate time each day to engage in activities that recharge and nourish your mind, body, and soul. This could include practicing mindfulness, taking a relaxing bath, reading a book, or pursuing a hobby that brings you joy.

3. Plan Balanced Meals: Create a meal plan that focuses on whole, nutritious foods. Include a variety of fruits, vegetables, lean proteins, whole grains, and healthy fats in your meals. Plan your meals in advance, prepare healthy snacks, and practice mindful eating to develop a positive relationship with food.
4. Schedule Exercise: Make physical activity a regular part of your day. Find activities that you enjoy and that align with your fitness goals. It could be as simple as taking a walk during your lunch break, practicing yoga in the morning, or engaging in a workout routine that suits your preferences and fitness level.
5. Manage Stress: Incorporate stress management techniques into your daily routine. Practice deep breathing exercises, engage in meditation or mindfulness practices, or find activities that help you relax and unwind. Prioritise activities that bring you joy and help you release stress.
6. Get Adequate Sleep: Create a bedtime routine that promotes quality sleep. Establish a consistent sleep schedule, create a sleep-friendly environment, and practice relaxation techniques before bed. Limit screen time and exposure to blue light and ensure your sleep environment is comfortable and conducive to restful sleep.
7. Seek Support: Surround yourself with a support system that encourages and supports your holistic wellness journey. Share your goals and progress with trusted friends or family members who can provide encouragement and accountability. Consider joining wellness communities. Consult with healthcare professionals, nutritionists, fitness trainers, or holistic wellness coaches who can provide expert advice and guidance. They can help

you assess your needs, develop a comprehensive plan, and offer ongoing support. Their expertise ensures that your plan is well-informed and tailored to your specific requirements.
8. Regularly Assess and Adjust: Continuously evaluate your holistic wellness plan to determine what is working well and what may need adjustment. Regularly assess your progress towards your goals, identify any obstacles, and make necessary tweaks to your plan. Stay open to new ideas and approaches that can enhance your overall well-being.

Getting down to the details

1. Set Realistic Goals: Define clear and achievable goals that align with your overall well-being. These goals should be specific, measurable, attainable, relevant, and time-bound (SMART). Consider both short-term and long-term goals, such as improving your diet, increasing physical activity, managing stress, or enhancing your sleep patterns. By setting realistic goals, you can track your progress and stay motivated on your wellness journey. For example, if your goal is to improve your nutrition, set specific targets such as eating a balanced breakfast every morning or incorporating more fruits and vegetables into your meals.
2. Identify Your Priorities: Determine which aspects of holistic wellness are most important to you. Everyone's priorities may differ based on their individual needs and values. For instance, if mental well-being is a priority, you may focus on mindfulness practices or seeking therapy. If physical fitness is your focus, you might emphasise regular exercise and healthy eating. Understanding your

priorities will help you allocate time and resources accordingly.
3. Customise Your Plan: Tailor your holistic wellness plan to fit your unique preferences, lifestyle, and circumstances. Consider factors such as your daily schedule, commitments, and resources available. Choose activities that you enjoy and can realistically incorporate into your routine. For example, if you prefer outdoor activities, you could include nature walks or outdoor yoga sessions. Personalising your plan increases the likelihood of adherence and long-term success.
4. Track Your Progress: Regularly monitor and evaluate your progress to stay motivated and adjust as needed. Keep a wellness journal or use digital tools to record your daily activities, thoughts, and feelings related to your holistic wellness journey. Celebrate your achievements, no matter how small, and learn from any setbacks. Tracking your progress helps you stay accountable and empowers you to make informed decisions for your well-being.
5. Adapt and Evolve: Recognise that your holistic wellness plan may need adjustments over time. Life, circumstances, goals, and priorities can change, so it's important to be flexible and willing to adapt. Regularly reassess your plan, reassess your goals, and make necessary modifications to ensure it remains aligned with your evolving needs and aspirations.

Creating a personalised holistic wellness plan is about finding what works for you and aligning it with your unique lifestyle. Adapt the techniques to fit your schedule, preferences, and needs. By creating a personalised holistic wellness plan that suits your lifestyle, you take an active role in nurturing your well-being. This tailored approach allows you to address your unique needs, find balance, and foster a sustainable and fulfilling way of living. Remember, it's a journey of self-discovery and continuous growth, so embrace the process and enjoy the positive impact it has on your overall health and happiness.

A system for implementing your short- and medium-term goals.

I came across this system contained in a book by Frederick Dodson in his book, 'Parallel Universes of Self.' A book I thoroughly recommend. This is a bullet point way of establishing 'the how' to fulfil your objectives. I apply this exercise ever since I first came upon it. It has provided a beacon of clarity in implementing and completing my goals. I trust it assists you in a similar way.

Parallel Universes Exercise

1. Create a list of your goals in writing. These can be short-term, medium-term, and long-term goals.
2. Choose the goal that shines brightest, evokes most interest, and the most energy regardless of its reasonableness. Interest and joy are reliable intuitive indicators of what is right for you.
3. Pursue that goal until it has used up all its energy.
4. Now you enter a new scenario.
5. From your short-, medium-, and long-term goals list, review and, if necessary, update.
6. Assess the available options, and now choose the new goal with the most energy and pursue it again to the best of your knowledge.
7. Again, when the goal seems fulfilled and loses energy, don't criticise yourself; instead, ask, 'Which goal, from my list, has the most energy now?'
8. There will always be an option that stands out and offers itself. Follow that new goal and repeat this process right through to until the end of your life.

9. By following this approach, you align with your soul's plan and accelerate your path to higher consciousness and the life experiences you intended to have.

Some suggestions for holistic health in daily action

1. Morning Rituals: Begin your day with intention by creating a morning ritual that sets a positive tone for the rest of the day. This could include activities such as meditation, gentle stretching, journaling, or affirmations. Take a few moments to centre yourself and cultivate a positive mindset before diving into your daily responsibilities.
2. Mindful Eating: Make mealtimes a ritual of nourishment and mindfulness. Sit down and savour your meals, paying attention to the flavours, textures, and nourishment they provide. Chew your food slowly, savouring each bite. Practice gratitude for the nourishment and energy it gives you.
3. Movement Breaks: Incorporate short movement breaks throughout your day to keep your body energised and reduce the negative effects of sedentary behaviour. Take a walk during your lunch break, stretch your muscles, or engage in a brief workout. Movement not only benefits your physical well-being but also helps boost your mood and productivity.
4. Self-Care Rituals: Carve out time each day for self-care activities that promote relaxation and rejuvenation. This could include taking a warm bath, practicing self-massage, reading a book, or engaging in a hobby you enjoy. Prioritise self-care as an essential part of your daily routine.
5. Technology Detox: Establish a ritual of unplugging from technology for a designated period each day.

Set boundaries around your device usage and create a technology-free zone or time. Use this opportunity to engage in activities that promote connection, such as spending quality time with loved ones, engaging in outdoor activities, or pursuing hobbies that don't involve screens.

6. Evening Wind-Down: Create an evening ritual to unwind and prepare your mind and body for restful sleep. This could involve practicing relaxation techniques, such as deep breathing or meditation, dimming the lights, reading a book, or engaging in a calming activity before bed. Disconnect from all electronic screens at least an hour before bedtime to promote better sleep quality.

7. Reflection and Gratitude: End each day with a moment of reflection and gratitude. Take a few minutes to journal or mentally reflect on the events of the day, acknowledging your achievements, challenges, and areas of growth. Cultivating a gratitude practice can help shift your focus towards the positive and foster a sense of contentment and appreciation.

8. Sleep Rituals: Establish a consistent bedtime routine that signals to your body it's time to unwind and prepare for sleep. This may include activities like practicing gentle stretches, drinking herbal tea, reading a book, or practicing relaxation exercises. Create a peaceful sleep environment by keeping the room cool, dark, and quiet.

9. Meditation practice, use technology to your advantage. Use phone applications for your meditation practice. Most can be used free of charge. Select the applications that you feel most at home with. There are a variety of different styles of meditation practice available, experiment and update your meditation applications to suit your

mood and interest.
10. Yoga and fitness phone applications are also available some free and some are subscription only. These are useful to experiment with before taking out membership with a gym or yoga classes. The decision to enrol in the gym should be confirmed by your own personal interest.
11. Having a journal of your body's statistics puts you in charge of your physical wellness records and is a great mood uplifter or a reminder to step up and do more. Google Fit is one the many free applications available that you can use to record your statistics. Google Fit enables you to record your heart points, daily steps, distance walked, minutes of movement, weight, energy expended in calories etc. There is also a very useful World Health Organisation supported statistic of Heart Points to be scored per week, the target is a minimum of 150 heart points per week. (You score Heart Points for each minute that gets your heart pumping, e.g., like a brisk walk. Increase the intensity to earn even more heart points.)
12. Invest in a smart watch which can keep you abreast of your state of fitness. To know your pulse rate, blood pressure, blood oxygen level, sleep, and daily step count are valuable indicators of wellness that you should be abreast of. Use these indicators to keep a 'finger on the pulse' of your body's working.
    a) Pulse – know your 'at rest' pulse rate and your maximum pulse rate when exercising vigorously.
    b) Blood pressure – take every week and keep records in your journal or fitness phone application.
    c) Blood oxygen levels – a good indicator that you are breathing in sufficient oxygen into

       d) Sleep – you should know your hours of sleep, the quality of your sleep, the ratio between deep sleep, REM sleep and light sleep. Sleep is a vital source of brain and body recharge, keep track of it. Some excellent phone applications will avail you of this information.

       e) Daily step count – an excellent way of gauging your daily walking exercise.

Establishing daily rituals is about finding practices that resonate with you and incorporating them into your routine with consistency. These rituals provide structure, grounding, and a sense of purpose, supporting your overall well-being. Customise your rituals based on your preferences and needs and allow them to evolve as you continue your holistic wellness journey.

Overcoming common challenges and obstacles

This requires consistent effort and a proactive mindset. Here are some practical day-to-day strategies you can apply to overcome these hurdles:

Overcome lack of Motivation

1. Set specific and achievable goals: Break down your larger wellness goals into smaller, manageable tasks. Celebrate each milestone you achieve to stay motivated.
2. Find inspiration: Surround yourself with motivational quotes, images, or stories that resonate with your wellness journey. Engage with uplifting content through books, podcasts, or online communities.
3. Seek support: Connect with like-minded individuals who share similar goals. Join wellness groups or find an accountability partner to keep each other

motivated and accountable.

Time Constraints

1. Prioritise self-care: Identify the activities that contribute most to your overall well-being and make them non-negotiable. Schedule time for exercise, meal preparation, mindfulness practices, or any other self-care activities that rejuvenate you.
2. Optimise your schedule: Evaluate your daily routine and identify areas where you can maximise efficiency. Look for time-saving strategies, such as combining exercise with commuting or incorporating mindfulness practices during breaks.

Self-Doubt and Negative Self-Talk

1. Practice self-compassion: Treat yourself with kindness and understanding. Embrace imperfections and learn from setbacks. Remind yourself of your strengths and achievements.
2. Challenge negative thoughts: Identify negative self-talk patterns and replace them with commitments for you to achieve. Focus on your progress and remind yourself of your potential for growth and success.
3. Surround yourself with positivity: Engage with uplifting and inspirational content, surround yourself with supportive people, and seek out mentors or coaches who can provide guidance and encouragement.

Plateaux and Setbacks

1. Embrace change and variety: Introduce new exercises, wellness practices, or healthy recipes to break through plateaux. Explore different

approaches to find what works best for you.
2. Reflect and adjust: When facing setbacks, take a step back to assess the situation. Reflect on what might have contributed to the setback and adjust your approach accordingly. Seek guidance from experts or mentors who can provide insights and help you navigate challenges.

Lack of Knowledge or Guidance

1. Educate yourself: Read books, attend workshops, or listen to podcasts on wellness-related topics. Follow reputable sources and stay informed about the latest research and practices.
2. Seek professional guidance: Consult experts in specific areas of wellness, such as nutritionists, fitness trainers, or therapists. Their expertise can provide valuable insights tailored to your unique needs.

Overwhelm and Stress

1. Practice stress management: Incorporate stress-reducing techniques into your daily routine, such as meditation, deep breathing exercises, or engaging in hobbies and activities you enjoy.
2. Prioritise self-care: Set aside dedicated time each day for self-care activities that help you relax and recharge. This could include taking a bath, reading a book, going for a walk-in nature, or practicing mindfulness.

Social and Environmental Factors

1. Communicate your needs: Clearly express your wellness goals and boundaries to your loved ones. Seek their understanding and support, and kindly ask them to respect your choices.

2. **Create an empowering environment:** Surround yourself with positive influences. Create a physical space that supports your wellness journey, such as keeping healthy snacks accessible or creating a dedicated exercise area at home.

Accountability and Consistency

1. **Track your progress:** Keep a journal or use mobile apps to monitor your activities, goals, and progress. Seeing your achievements visually can boost motivation and accountability.
2. **Find an accountability partner:** Pair up with a friend, family member, or colleague who shares similar wellness goals. Regularly check in with each other, provide support, and hold each other accountable.

Overcoming challenges is a continuous process. By implementing these practical strategies into your daily life, you can navigate obstacles with resilience, maintain momentum, and achieve lasting wellness success.

Here are ways to sustain long-term holistic wellness practices for reaping the full benefits and enjoying a balanced and fulfilling life. Consistency is Key

1. **Establish routines:** Incorporate wellness activities into your daily schedule. Whether it's a morning meditation, an evening walk, or regular healthy meal preparation, make them non-negotiable parts of your day.
2. **Set reminders:** Use alarms, calendar notifications, or mobile apps to remind you of your wellness practices. These gentle nudges can help you stay on track and prioritise self-care.

Reflect and Celebrate

1. Regular self-assessment: Take time to reflect on your progress and the positive changes you've experienced. Assess what's working well and areas that may need adjustment.
2. Celebrate milestones: Acknowledge and celebrate your achievements along the way. This can reinforce your commitment to holistic wellness and motivate you to continue your journey.

Find Joy in the Process

1. Discover what you love: Engage in activities that bring you joy and align with your wellness goals. Whether it's dancing, painting, playing a musical instrument, or practicing yoga, find what resonates with you and make it a part of your regular routine.
2. Seek new experiences: Embrace opportunities to try new things. Explore different forms of exercise, mindfulness practices, or wellness modalities to keep your routine fresh and exciting.

Surround Yourself with Support

1. Connect with a community: Join wellness groups, online forums, or local meetups to connect with like-minded individuals who share similar goals. Surrounding yourself with a supportive community can provide encouragement, inspiration, and accountability.
2. Share your journey: Openly discuss your holistic wellness practices with your friends, family, or colleagues. By sharing your experiences, you may inspire others to embark on their own wellness journeys and receive support in return.

Adapt and Evolve

1. Embrace flexibility: Understand that life is dynamic, and your wellness practices may need adjustments at different stages. Be open to adapting your routines, exploring new techniques, and refining your approach to fit your changing needs.
2. Continual learning: Stay curious and seek out new knowledge about holistic wellness. Read books, attend workshops, or listen to podcasts to expand your understanding and incorporate fresh ideas into your practices.

Practice Self-Compassion

1. Embrace imperfections: Understand that wellness is a lifelong journey with ups and downs. Be kind to yourself and embrace self-compassion during challenging times.
2. Learn from setbacks: View setbacks as learning opportunities rather than failures. Analyse what triggered the setback and use it as a stepping stone for growth and resilience.

Dear Reader, I offer you a final inspiring thought from the author, Graham Anderson,

"Do something for the world so fantastic that it changes the world for the benefit of humanity. Every change so far has been made by ordinary people. Thus, the trick is not to limit your beliefs."

Enjoy the possibilities.

GERARD ANTHONY LANKESTER

Mastering Holistic Wellness,
A Practical Guide for Every Day.

APPENDIX 1 - MY CURRENT DAILY ROUTINE

Daily Routine

1. Sleep routine. Up at 05.00 daily and in bed for 21.30 to 22.00 daily. My smart watch measures my sleeping pattern, in addition, I use the phone application, Sleep Tracker, to monitor hours slept, together with a breakdown between light sleep, deep sleep and REM sleep.
2. Meditation 1 hour plus daily. I use a mixture of breathing exercises as well as the following phone applications for guided meditations.
    a) Healthy Minds Programme – I have used now for around 4 or 5 years. An excellent programme. It takes around 9 months to complete the course at the rate of one section per day. The application is free.
    b) Serenity – Excellent short daily meditation, lasting 3 minutes. The short meditations are free, the longer ones by subscription.
    c) Insight Timer – Excellent variety of meditations to select from daily. You can check in daily on your mood to identify what and why you feel as you do. I use the free application, though extended courses are by

subscription.
d) Let's Meditate – a good range of short and extended meditations. Updated periodically also. Free application.
e) I update my choices of phone applications to use if I feel the interest wanes. There are a wide range to choose from on Samsung App Store.

3) Reading 1 hour plus daily. I use the Kindle Unlimited subscription service. This enables me to take out up to 20 books at a time to read. I usually have eight books on the go at any one time. I find the Kindle algorithm of great help to identify books around a chosen subject. I tend to read non-fiction subjects. I read one chapter from each of the books I have subscribed to, each day. It allows me to encompass a wide range of topics every day.

4) Exercise is critical, and I exercise daily for 60 to 120 minutes. My principal choice is brisk walking. I also have an exercise bike to enable me to practice HIIT training, twice weekly. I also have a cross trainer for use for when the rain prevents walking outdoors. I also keep a set of weights to maintain muscle mass. I use the Google Fit application to monitor Heart Points, steps walked, weight, energy expended. This application is so useful for keeping your finger on the pulse of your exercise regime. In addition, I use a smart watch to measure heat rate and once a week take a Blood Pressure reading all are recorded on the Google Fit application.

5) Nutrition - I am a pescatarian who has kept to a low carbohydrate food plan regime for many years.

6) I weigh all foods to be consumed and monitor and log on a phone application, My Net Diary. This application is great for monitoring calorie intake, the mix between Carbohydrates, Protein and Fats. Saturated Fat intake, sodium, dietary Fibre and Calcium. It is available as a free application. The Premium service offers more

detailed analysis of vitamin and nutrient intake. There is another excellent application called Nutracheck that has similar functions.

7) Following a test at a dietician I discovered that I have an intolerance to wheat so avoid all wheat and wheat flour products.
8) I avoid all starchy carbohydrate foods and sugar.
9) I make my own fermented foods – sauerkraut and kefir.
10) I took up intermittent fasting a couple of years ago. I operate a 16/8 fasting/eating window. From 08.00 to 16.00 eating window. 16.00 to 08.00 fasting window. I use the phone application, Fasting Tracker, to monitor progress.

This regime enables me to maintain an informed view of my progress in maintaining Holistic Wellness.

GERARD ANTHONY LANKESTER

Mastering Holistic Wellness,
A Practical Guide for Every Day.

ACKNOWLEDGEMENTS

My thanks to my family and friends for their encouragement and support. This book has been many years in its gestation, and I am elated that the information is now available in one volume for the world to read.

My sincere thanks also go to Haus of Ra for the excellent photographic work on the front and back covers of this book.

COPYRIGHT

Gerard Anthony Lankester has asserted his right to be identified as the author of this work in accordance with the Copyright, Designs and Patents Act of 1988. All rights reserved.

No part of this publication may be reproduced, stored in a retrieval system, or transmitted in any form or by any means, electronic, mechanical, photocopying, recording, or otherwise, without the prior permission of both the copyright owner and the publisher of this book.

DISCLAIMER

The content and ideas presented in "Mastering Holistic Wellness: A Practical Guide for Every Day" are the result of the collaborative efforts between the author and the AI language model. While the AI model has been trained on a diverse range of data sources, the specific attributions for the content generated by the language model are not available. Therefore, the information provided in the book should be used as a general guide and readers are encouraged to consult additional sources for a comprehensive understanding of holistic wellness. The AI-generated elements in the book have been reviewed and edited by the author to align with their expertise and vision.

THE BEST WAY TO ACHIEVE

Mental Holistic Wellness

is to take

"radical responsibility"

for every aspect of your

mind, body, and spiritual

well-being.

Gerard Anthony Lankester

Printed in Great Britain
by Amazon